T0309980

Intelligent Bioinformatics

Intelligent Bioinformatics

The application of artificial intelligence techniques to bioinformatics problems

Edward Keedwell
and
Ajit Narayanan

School of Engineering, Computer Science and Mathematics
University of Exeter, UK

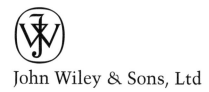

John Wiley & Sons, Ltd

Copyright © 2005   John Wiley & Sons Ltd, The Atrium, Southern Gate, Chichester,
West Sussex PO19 8SQ, England

Telephone   (+44) 1243 779777

Email (for orders and customer service enquiries): cs-books@wiley.co.uk
Visit our Home Page on www.wileyeurope.com or www.wiley.com

Reprinted 2006

All Rights Reserved. No part of this publication may be reproduced, stored in a retrieval
system or transmitted in any form or by any means, electronic, mechanical, photocopying,
recording, scanning or otherwise, except under the terms of the Copyright, Designs and
Patents Act 1988 or under the terms of a licence issued by the Copyright Licensing Agency
Ltd, 90 Tottenham Court Road, London W1T 4LP, UK, without the permission in writing of
the Publisher. Requests to the Publisher should be addressed to the Permissions Department,
John Wiley & Sons Ltd, The Atrium, Southern Gate, Chichester, West Sussex PO19 8SQ,
England, or emailed to permreq@wiley.co.uk, or faxed to (+44) 1243 770620.

Designations used by companies to distinguish their products are often claimed as trademarks.
All brand names and product names used in this book are trade names, service marks,
trademarks or registered trademarks of their respective owners. The Publisher is not
associated with any product or vendor mentioned in this book.

This publication is designed to provide accurate and authoritative information in regard to
the subject matter covered. It is sold on the understanding that the Publisher is not engaged
in rendering professional services. If professional advice or other expert assistance is
required, the services of a competent professional should be sought.

Other Wiley Editorial Offices

John Wiley & Sons Inc., 111 River Street, Hoboken, NJ 07030, USA

Jossey-Bass, 989 Market Street, San Francisco, CA 94103-1741, USA

Wiley-VCH Verlag GmbH, Boschstr. 12, D-69469 Weinheim, Germany

John Wiley & Sons Australia Ltd, 33 Park Road, Milton, Queensland 4064, Australia

John Wiley & Sons (Asia) Pte Ltd, 2 Clementi Loop #02-01, Jin Xing Distripark,
Singapore 129809

John Wiley & Sons Canada Ltd, 22 Worcester Road, Etobicoke, Ontario, Canada M9W 1L1

Wiley also publishes its books in a variety of electronic formats. Some content that appears
in print may not be available in electronic books.

Library of Congress Cataloguing-in-Publication Data

British Library Cataloguing in Publication Data

A catalogue record for this book is available from the British Library

ISBN 10: 0 470 02175 6 (HB)   ISBN 13: 978 0 470 02175 0 (HB)

Typeset in 10.5/13.5pt Sabon by TechBooks, New Delhi, India
Printed and bound in Great Britain by TJ International Ltd., Padstow, Corwall
This book is printed on acid-free paper responsibly manufactured from sustainable forestry
in which at least two trees are planted for each one used for paper production.

Contents

Preface

It is widely recognized that the field of biology is in the midst of a 'data explosion'. A series of technical advances in recent years has increased the amount of data that biologists can record about different aspects of an organism at the genomic, transcriptomic and proteomic levels. This data is, of course, vital to advancing our knowledge. In recent years, the discipline of *bioinformatics* has allowed biologists to make full use of the advances in computer science and computational statistics in analysing this data. However, as the volume of data grows, the techniques used must become more sophisticated to cater for large-scale data and noise. Also, given the growth in biological data, there is a need to extract information that was not previously known from these databases to supplement current knowledge. Large databases may contain interesting patterns that, if identified and authenticated by further laboratory and clinical work, can lead to novel theories about the causes of various diseases and also possibly to new drugs for their treatment. The discipline of bioinformatics has reached the end of its first phase, and the motivation behind this book is to characterize the principles that may underlie second phase bioinformatics. That is, second phase bioinformatics is when the discipline, instead of being informed by just computer science and computational statistics, is also informed by artificial intelligence techniques.

As we show in this book, there are problems in bioinformatics and many other sciences that cannot be solved satisfactorily even with the fastest computers. Clearly, a more 'intelligent' approach is required to solve these increasingly difficult bioinformatics problems, such as gene expression analysis and protein structure prediction. This book attempts to address this by looking at the latest advances in artificial intelligence technology as applied to computational problems in biology. Artificial intelligence methods are often based on the ways in which humans solve search and optimization problems, or how nature has solved its own problems, for example by using the principles of 'survival of the fittest' in evolutionary computation.

This book is divided into three parts, each containing a number of chapters. These parts are designed to allow readers to access the material most relevant to them. The first part, *Introduction,* introduces the material necessary to understand the technology and biology included in the later chapters. We recognize that bioinformatics is highly cross-disciplinary and therefore some, all or none of these chapters may be relevant to the reader, depending on their background. The next part, *Current Techniques,* describes the established artificial intelligence techniques in bioinformatics including probabilistic, nearest neighbour and genetic algorithm approaches. The final part, *Future Techniques,* is intended to give the reader an impression of the latest thinking in the area of intelligent bioinformatics. Some of these approaches may not have been widely applied to problems in bioinformatics, but algorithms such as genetic programming and various hybrid approaches can be expected to make a big impact in this domain if experience in other areas of science and technology is anything to go by.

In short, this book has been written to engage and interest readers from many disciplines. Biologists are provided for in that there is a full introduction to the challenges for computer science, and computer scientists should also find the chapters on biology and bioinformatics informative. Practicing bioinformaticians are also likely to find the book enlightening, as much of the material has previously only been included in specialist publications and a collection such as this provides a single resource for many intelligent problem-solving techniques in bioinformatics. However, as with any book of this type, not every technique can be included due to space restrictions and apologies are offered to researchers whose own favourite analytical techniques are not covered in this book.

Edward Keedwell
Ajit Narayanan

Acknowledgements

The authors would like to thank everyone involved with producing this book including staff at the Department of Computer Science and Centre for Water Systems at the University of Exeter, in particular Godfrey Walters, Dragan Savic and Soon-Thiam Khu. In addition to this, we would like to thank Bjorn Olsson for his contribution to the tutorials on which this book is based, and Laetitia Jourdan for her helpful comments. Also, we would like to thank the many MSc students on the Bioinformatics programme at the University of Exeter, who contributed towards some of the material for this book. Finally we would also like to thank the editorial and production staff at Wiley, in particular Joan Marsh, Andrea Baier and Robert Hambrook for making this book possible.

We are grateful to WoltersKluwer Health for permission to adapt and re-use Figures 2.10, 6.3, 7.1, 7.2 and 7.3 and Table 5.1 from 'Artificial intelligence techniques for bioinformatics', A. Narayanan, E. C. Keedwell and B. Olsson, *Applied Bioinformatics* 2002: 1(4) 191–222.

Dedications

Ed Keedwell – This book is dedicated to my family Rob, Lyn, Rich and Loveday, to Kate, and in memory of Alex Larigo.

Ajit Narayanan – This book is dedicated to Lucy, Belinda and Kieran, my mother Janaki, my brother Ramesh and sister Seetha.

Part 1
Introduction

1
Introduction to the Basics of Molecular Biology

1.1 Basic cell architecture

A cell, typically 10–30 millionths of a metre (10–30μm) across for humans, contains many specialized structures called *organelles* (Figure 1.1). The *cell membrane* controls the passage of substances into and out of the cell and encloses cell organelles as well as cell substances; the *cytoplasm* serves as a fluid container for cell organelles and other cell substances as well as helping in the transport of substances within the cell; the *nucleus* directs all cell activity and carries hereditary information; the *endoplasmic reticulum* serves as a transport network and storage area for substances within the cell; the *ribosome* manufactures different kinds of cell protein; the *Golgi apparatus* packages protein for storage or transport out of the cell; the *lysosome* digests or breaks down food materials into simpler parts and removes waste materials from the cell; the *mitochondria* serve as the power supply of the cell by producing ATP – adenosine triphosphate – which is the source of energy for all cell activities; *microtubules* serve as the support system or skeleton of the cell; and *microfilaments* assist in cell motility. Each organelle performs one or more special task(s) to keep the cell alive.

In addition to this *intracellular* (within cell) architecture, there is also an *intercellular* (between cell) architecture: cells form tissue (aggregations of similar cells that perform some subfunction), which in turn combines with other tissues to form organs (aggregation of subfunctions to perform

Intelligent Bioinformatics   Edward Keedwell and Ajit Narayanan
© 2005 John Wiley & Sons, Ltd

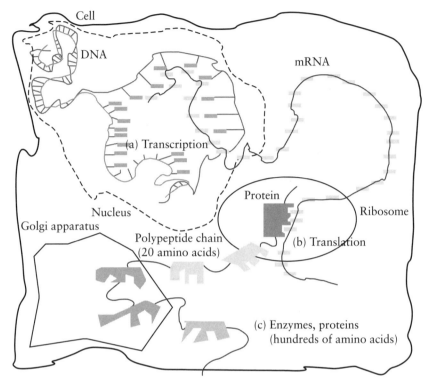

Figure 1.1   An overview of a typical human cell

an overall function), which in turn together form an organism (aggregation of all functions to keep the multicellular organism alive). The rest of
this chapter deals with just two of these organelles, the nucleus and the
ribosomes, and the processes within a cell that links them together.

1.2 The structure, content and scale
of deoxyribonucleic acid (DNA)

DNA and chromosomes

All the information directing every cell function is stored in large DNA
molecules found in the nucleus. A cell cannot function without DNA.
The information it contains must somehow be made available to the rest
of the cell as well as being passed on to all new cells. Although each
cell contains the full complement of DNA, through some process which
is not yet clearly understood certain parts of the DNA are switched on

or off within cells, resulting in different types of cell producing different proteins for normal growth and functioning of the organism as a whole.

The human body consists of between 30 to 80 trillion cells, where one trillion $= 10^{12}$, i.e. one thousand billion, where one billion equals one thousand million. What is shown in Figure 1.1 is a eukaryote cell, which has a membrane-bound nucleus. The human body has about 200 different types of eukaryote cell. The process of *transcription* (Figure 1.1(a)) starts with the double-stranded DNA opening up to reveal bases coding for a gene. A copy of the gene is made called messenger RNA (mRNA) which leaves the nucleus. The double-stranded DNA closes after transcription. At ribosomes, the process of *translation* starts (Figure 1.1(b)) whereby three copied bases at a time (codon) are mapped onto one amino acid. The mRNA is broken up and may re-enter the nucleus for further mRNA transcription. The growing sequence of amino acids (polypeptide sequence) may be amended by the Golgi apparatus before the final production of enzymes, proteins and other translated products (Figure 1.1 (c)).

The DNA in the nucleus takes the form of large molecules called *chromosomes* made up of combinations of four types of nucleotides – adenine, guanine, thymine and cytosine (labelled 'A', 'G', 'T' and 'C', respectively). Chromosomal structure can be described at different levels. At the lowest level, single strands of DNA are paired with their complementary bases to form double strands (about two billionths of a metre ($2\eta m$) wide). These double strands form strings of *chromatin* about $11\eta m$ wide that are packed tightly into $30\eta m$-wide chromatin fibre. Chromatin fibre is itself densely packed into a section of chromosome about $300\eta m$ wide which again is packed into condensed sections of chromosome about $700\eta m$ wide. Finally, chromosome sections are joined together at the *centromere* to form an entire chromosome about $1400\eta m$ ($1.4\mu m$, or 0.0014mm) wide.

The extreme small scale of DNA and its structure means that it cannot be observed directly. Since the largest magnification that can be seen through an optical microscope is $400\times$ and the closest that two distinct spots can be resolved is 0.2 mm, if a chromosome can be seen at all through an optical microscope using artificial or natural light it will be as a fuzzy image. Lightwaves with shorter wavelengths (such as blue or ultraviolet) can be used to increase resolution (the resolution limit is about 0.45 times the wavelength), but then special techniques are required to capture the image, since such short wavelengths are beyond visual capability. Light microscopy can be used to observe a cell but still cannot make out the organelles with clarity. One of the most popular techniques is *transmission electron microscopy* (TEM), where electrons are beamed through the sample and an image produced resulting from the interaction of the electrons with the sample. TEM can resolve organelles and other subcellular structures but not the content of chromosomes. In other words, it is likely that chromosome content will not be observed directly at the level of bases, which means that DNA sequences will never be observed directly. Instead, *indirect* methods for observing and measuring DNA must be used.

It is estimated that the DNA in each human cell contains about six or seven billion nucleotides, spread across 46 chromosomes (discrete molecular structures of DNA), each one of which takes the shape of a double helix. If all the DNA in one cell were stretched end to end, the length is estimated to be about 2 m. That is, each DNA chromosome is about 50 000 times shorter than its extended length.

Nucleotides are conventionally portrayed as shapes that lock onto each other when paired on the two strands that make up the double-helix structure of a chromosome. Complementary base pairing is represented in Figure 1.2(a) and (b), with T on one strand always being paired with A on the other strand, and C with G. Each strand has directionality (the direction in which nucleotides code for genes), known as 5′ (5-prime) or 3′. That is, the strands run in the opposite direction to each other and are 'anti-parallel'. In Figure 1.2(c), the nucleotides making up a gene have a direction from the 5′ to the 3′ end (left-to-right for the 'top' strand,

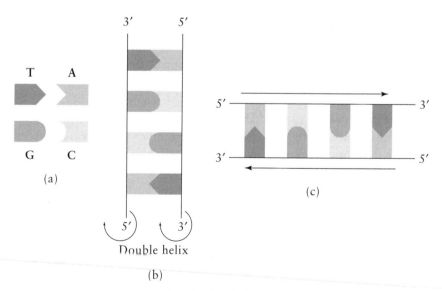

Figure 1.2   The double-helix structure

right-to-left for the 'bottom' strand). Each nucleotide is a molecule consisting of a five-carbon sugar (deoxyribose for DNA), a phosphate group, and a nitrogenous base (a ring compound containing nitrogen), with each carbon being given a number $1'$ to $5'$. Nucleotides form a chain when phosphodiester linkages are formed between the sugar portions of the molecules. As a result of the phosphates being linked from the $5'$ carbon on one sugar to the $3'$ carbon on the next, the DNA sequence has a free $5'$ carbon (no nucleotide attached) at one end and a free $3'$ carbon at the other end. These free carbon numbers are then used to signify the directionality of the sequence.

Types of cell

Eukaryotic cells mainly appear in multicellular organisms (e.g. plants, animals) and are distinguished by having a clearly designated nucleus containing DNA structured into chromosomes, while *prokaryotic* cells (single cell organisms) have no such nucleus and their DNA is stored in one, usually circular, molecule. Prokaryotic cells are usually called *bacteria* and represent the simplest life forms. There are three classes of bacteria. *Eubacteria* are the most common type and can cause disease in humans either by directly producing toxins harmful to us or by being infected by bacterial viruses that then cause the bacteria in us to produce harmful toxins. In addition to the trillions of eukaryotic cells that make up a human, human bodies also tolerate a large number of bacteria that produce useful proteins, e.g. for breaking down some types of food, that human DNA could not otherwise manufacture. *Archaebacteria* are typically found in hostile (usually hot, acidic and oxygenless) environments and are assumed to be, or descended from, among the oldest living organisms on this planet, since the early Earth would not have contained oxygen and would have been a hot place. *Cyanobacteria* use photosynthesis (the process of converting energy in sunlight into chemicals used by living systems) and are believed to be the source of chloroplasts in plants. The remainder of this book will concentrate on eukaryotic cells, such as those found in multicellular creatures.

The human body is made up of large numbers of about 200 different types of eukaryotic cell, such as nerve cells (neurons) for communication and control, muscle cells for producing mechanical force, and sensory cells such as those in the eye and skin. Since all humans (and other multicellular organisms) start as one fertilized egg cell, it is one of the mysteries of modern biology as to why, after division like a prokaryotic cell, the subsequent cells remain together to cooperate for further division and specialization into all of the different types of cell, until a full-grown human develops. Most prokaryotic cells, after division, go their own way and lead independent lives.

DNA, the genome and genes

For human and other eukaryotic cells, two polynucleotide chains (that is, two sequences consisting of many different occurrences of the four neucleotides) form the DNA double helix, with all the bases on the inside of the helix and the sugar-phosphate backbones on the outside (Figure 1.2). Under normal cellular conditions, adenine and guanine (*purines*) always pair with thymine and cytosine (*pyramidines*), respectively and vice versa. The complete set of DNA in an organism's cell is its *genome*. A eukaryotic nucleus contains a number of chromosomes, each of which is a double-helix containing hundreds of thousands of bases on anti-parallel strands. In other words, while the strands are parallel in a chromosome, they run in an opposite direction to each other. One strand is read from 'left-to-right', or 'top-to-bottom', and its complement is read from 'right-to-left', or 'bottom-to-top'.

So far, the assumption is that a eukaryotic cell contains the full set of chromosomes, and this is true for about 99.99 per cent of all cells in the human body. However, before a normal eukaryotic cell can come into being it has to be created. A sex cell for humans contains 23 chromosomes, consisting of about 3.5 billion bases in total. A sex cell (haploid) is different from a normal cell in that it contains only half the complement of chromosomes required to form a normal (diploid cell). Only when two sex cells merge will a normal cell consisting of 46 chromosomes result. A sex cell for goldfish contains 47 chromosomes (94 chromosomes for a normal goldfish cell), for rice 12, for a fruit fly four, for a guinea pig 32.

A *gene* is defined to be a sequence of DNA or bases that code for a specific function/protein. However, a gene can have more than one form or version. So, while there may be a gene for, say, producing hair of a certain colour (a gross oversimplification), that gene will have different *alleles*, such as producing brown hair or blonde hair. A gene is like a variable that can take different values, to use a computational metaphor. It is not known for sure how many human genes are capable of having different allelic values or how many different allelic values exist for those genes that can vary. Some of these differences in allelic values are strongly associated with diseases, such as one particular type of diabetes where a gene which contributes to the production of insulin for breaking down glucose in the blood has a different form to the normal form or version of the gene. Other differences in allelic values provide normal variation between individuals' however. It is difficult to identify a genuine allelic difference when comparing the same gene across two individuals; the difference can be just one base in a multithousand-base gene sequence. Since the content of genes cannot be observed directly, only indirect ways of identifying differences between individuals for the same gene can be used, which leads to problems of knowing where the differences may be and finding methods for checking for the existence of these differences.

As stated earlier it is estimated that there are several trillion (between 30 trillion and 80 trillion) cells in the human body (for skin, muscles, liver, blood, heart, brain, etc.). Each such cell contains the full set of 46 chromosomes inherited from the mother and father (23 in each case, via sex cells). It is also estimated that one set of 23 chromosomes code for about 30 000 genes for humans. On average, about 100 000–150 000 bases are required for coding a gene, although this figure varies greatly from a few hundred to a few hundred thousand. Several thousand genes will on average reside on each chromosome. A *genome* is defined to be the complete set of chromosomes inherited from one parent.

1.3 History of the human genome

The task of sequencing all the bases of the human genome is called the *human genome project*, which originated in the early 1980s with Gen-Bank when US Department of Energy technicians entered sequences of As, Gs, Cs and Ts from journals into databases using special keyboards. New protocols subsequently allowed researchers to enter sequences via telephone, and later GenBank was transferred to the National Institute for Biotechnology Information (NCBI). In 1990, the Human Genome Project (HGP) was launched as a publicly-funded consortium consisting of four large sequencing centres in the USA, the Sanger Centre in Cambridge, UK, and various laboratories in Japan, France, Germany and China. Before the project was completed, in Spring 2000 Celera Genomics announced that they had a complete draft of the human genome. While the HGP adopted a systematic method for 'sequencing' (identifying the nucleotides along all the chromosomes of) the human genome section by section, Celera adopted a 'shotgun' approach, whereby they fragmented the genome into small, easily sequenced stretches and then reconstructed the genome through proprietary algorithms. Increases in computational power through the 1990s made Celera's approach possible. Celera used just one anonymous person's DNA, whereas the HGP required cross-checking with several people's DNA. Also, Celera repeated the sequencing three times, whereas HGP required more repetitions.

Initially and during the early 1990s, it was thought that the HGP would find 80 000 genes. As the HGP progressed, this figure was revised down to 20 000 to 30 000 genes. A rough calculation indicates that, if there are 3.5 billion bases on 23 chromosomes and 30 000 genes, then about 120 000 bases are required per gene on average. However, it is now estimated that 98–99 per cent of DNA in humans is 'redundant' (does not code for any function). Also, it is estimated that up to 99.9 per cent of one person's genes match another random person's perfectly. That is, any two people taken at random share the very same DNA sequence (allelic values) for nearly every single one of their genes, but the remaining 0.1 per cent vary. If 30 000 genes are assumed, then 0.1 per cent is 30, that is, there are still over a billion ways ($2^{30} = 1\,073\,741\,824$) that two people can differ from each other. This is assuming that each gene has a binary function (on/off, high/low, dark/fair, etc), whereas genes can be expected to be multivariate (take many values). For instance, if there are on average three different forms for each gene, there are still over 205 billion ways that two people can differ from each other, more than enough to code for a difference between any two humans currently living (the world's population is currently estimated to be about six billion). Also, if the estimate of how many genes humans share identically with each other is just a fraction lower, say 99.8 per cent, then there is even more genetic variability possible. These differences between values for a specific gene are called *polymorphisms* and the physical location of a specific gene on chromosomes is called its *locus*.

There is also increasing interest in the 'redundant' or 'junk' DNA, that is, DNA which is believed not to code for any protein. It is not clear whether such sections of DNA are the remains of previously useful DNA that now have no function, or whether non-coding DNA provides a structural aid to help stabilize chromosomes and the nucleus.

1.4 Genes and proteins

Genes code for various products that are used by the cells making up the tissue of the organism. These products are called *proteins* and they have two primary functions: *structural*, such as helping to form muscle, hair and microtubules, and *enzymatic*, such as the production of enzymes for starting various chemical reactions in the cell. Proteins therefore contribute to biological structure and function. Proteins also have three other functions: they can carry signals, they can transport molecules such as oxygen and they can regulate cell processes, such as defence mechanisms. The process by which genes are made into proteins is started by *RNA polymerase* coming into contact with a chromosome and identifying the start point of a gene. These molecules open up the double helix structure to expose the DNA strand making up the gene, and a complementary copy of the gene is made in the direction in which the gene is meant to be read. The process of copying genes into mRNA is called *transcription*, and the process of converting the mRNA into protein is called *translation*.

Transcription starts with the double-helix unwinding Figure 1.3(a) and exposing bases that represent the start of a gene. mRNA is then formed, whereby a complementary copy of the gene is made. Since transcription proceeds in the 3′ to 5′ direction (more details follow later), the mRNA has opposite 'polarity', that is, the start of the gene is now at the 5′ end of the mRNA (Figure 1.3(b)). *Introns*, or parts of the gene that do not code for a protein, are removed, typically by the mRNA folding over itself and forming loops that are cut off, leaving *exons* in the transcript. These transcripts containing exons only can be further edited (Figure 1.3(c)) so that alternative splice pathways for the same gene are formed, i.e. one gene can give rise to many different transcripts.

Transcription

The *transcription* process consists of three stages: initiation, elongation and termination. Regions of DNA which signal *initiation* are termed *promoters* and lie 'upstream' of the start of the actual gene (Figure 1.4). Initiation starts with molecules such as polymerase II enzymes finding promoter regions upstream (towards the 3′ end of a strand) of a gene. These regions consists of specific patterns of bases, known as the **CAAT** box and **TATA** box. The start point of a gene is typically 25 bases downstream of the **TATA** box for eukaryotes. It is believed that there are two regions of promoters. RNA polymerase II enzymes scan the helix looking for these regions and, when found, bind tightly to the region further away from the initiation point. The enzyme then binds to the second region closer to the start point and opens up the helix while at the same time releasing a factor which signals that mRNA should be formed. *Elongation* is the process by which an mRNA copy of the genetic information is

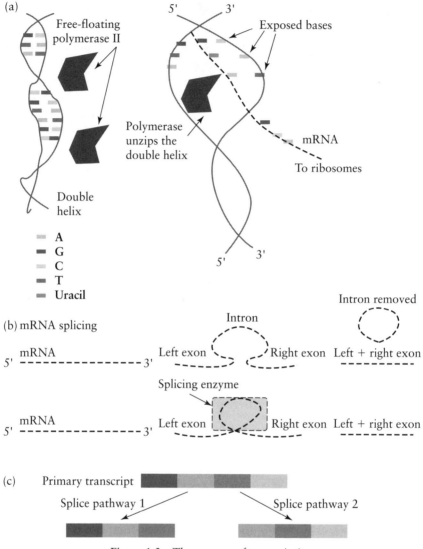

Figure 1.3   The process of transcription

actually made on the unravelled stretch of helix. Certain sequences may cause a pause during this process. *Termination* is caused in one of two ways. The first is a repeated sequence of bases that causes the mRNA to fold over itself and therefore terminate the transcription process. Typically, a **GC**-rich (guanine followed by cytosine) sequence is sufficient to terminate transcription. The second way is for a terminating factor to be released.

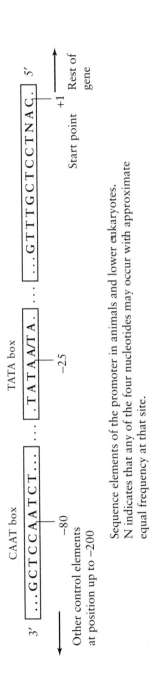

CAAT box

3′ | ...GCTCCAATCT... |

−80

Other control elements at position up to −200

TATA box

| ...TATAA/TA. |

−25

| ...GTTTGCTCCTNAC. | 5′

+1

Start point

Rest of gene

Sequence elements of the promoter in animals and lower eukaryotes. N indicates that any of the four nucleotides may occur with approximate equal frequency at that site.

Figure 1.4 The initiation stage

The process of transcription therefore results in a *complementary* copy of the gene, but there is one complication. C (cytosine) in DNA is transcribed as G (guanine), and G as C. However, while A (adenine) is transcribed to T (thymine), T is not transcribed to A. Instead, for transcription, a fifth base called *uracil* or *uradine* (U), which is functionally identical to adenine (A), is used. Faithful complementary base copying is used instead for another process, *replication*, whereby the entire genetic material of a cell is copied for cell division and the production of a new copy of the cell (*cloning*), such as when a new skin cell is required from an existing skin cell. Transcription therefore differs from replication in that transcription involves the use of a fifth base, uracil, which is the complementary base to adenine (A). U does not occur in replicated DNA, and T does not occur in mRNA.

As previously mentioned, at each nucleotide position along the double-stranded DNA molecule, the nucleotides are complementary. This is because, chemically, A forms two hydrogen bonds with T and C forms three hydrogen bonds with G. There is, however, a peculiar relationship between the directionality of DNA strands and the type of strand involved. One of the strands holds the information that represents a gene. This strand is called the *template* or *antisense* strand (containing *anti-codons*, to be described below). The other strand is called, confusingly, the *coding* or *sense* strand. The 'sense' and 'anti-sense' strands represent the two strands of the double helix (Figure 1.5). Transcription uses the anti-sense, or template, strand. Note that in replication a faithful copy of the sense strand produces the anti-sense strand with appropriate direction, and vice versa. The sense strand can therefore be regarded as containing 'DNA codons' (to be described later), and the anti-sense strand 'DNA anti-codons'. DNA codons and anti-codons are not to be confused with mRNA codons, which result from the transcription of the template strand

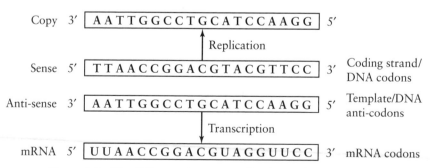

Figure 1.5   The difference between replication and transcription

and use U rather than T. There are therefore three ways that a gene can be described: through the template or antisense strand, through the coding or sense strand, and through the mRNA that is transcribed from the template or antisense strand.

Spliceosome and transcriptome

Just because a gene has been transcribed into mRNA does not mean that the task of making a copy of a gene has finished. Genes contain 'coding' and 'non-coding' regions. These regions are different from the 'junk DNA' mentioned earlier, which refers to the DNA between genes rather than within a gene. A coding region in a gene is that sequence of nucleotides within a gene that is actually used for making a protein. Even within a gene there are non-coding regions – nucleotide sequences that are not used for making a protein. These non-coding regions have to be removed from the mRNA, which is nothing but a faithful copy of a gene from beginning to end, including non-coding regions. After the mRNA has been 'edited' to remove introns, there is still another process that is only recently being understood. The remaining exons in the mRNA can themselves be 'edited' so that some exons are removed (Figure 1.3(b)) or shuffled to form alternative 'splice pathways' (that is, alternative ways that the remaining coding regions make up the final mRNA, Figure 1.3(c)). The study of how mRNA is formed from genes is called 'transcriptomics' and the total set of mRNA transcripts is called the 'transcriptome'. The transcriptome provides information as to which genes are being transcribed and which are not, depending on the cell type and various conditions experienced by the cell. The study of how mRNA is edited after initial transcription is called 'spliceosomics' and the total set of alternative splice pathways for all genes is called the 'spliceosome'. Recent advances in microarray technology have made transcriptomics and spliceosomics possible, as will be seen later.

There is growing interest in those regions of DNA within a gene which indicate exon/intron boundaries to try to understand the transcriptome in more detail. Introns, for eukaryotes including humans, average in length from about 200 to 400 nucleotides, but this figure can vary greatly (from 50 to about 30 000). Some of the longer introns may contain other genes, each with their own introns. Analysis of exon/intron boundaries reveals, with very few exceptions, a GT/AG rule, whereby the occurrence of GT towards the 5' end of a DNA sequence indicates the start of an intron and the occurrence of AG towards the 3' end indicates the end of the intron. It appears that internal splicing mechanisms recognize the mRNA counterparts to these duplets and remove the intervening sequence from the transcribed mRNA (called 'pre-mRNA'). Interest is also growing in alternative splicing models that capture alternative pathways for the removal of introns. Any DNA segment can therefore be an exon or an intron, depending on whether it is retained or removed during processing of pre-mRNA. Once all editing has taken place, the result is 'mature mRNA' which is ready for translation into a polypeptide chain.

Translation and the proteome

The mature mRNA leaves the nucleus and is transported to *ribosomes*, where translation into proteins takes place with the help of transfer RNA (tRNA). The nucleotides of the mRNA enter the ribosome sequentially from beginning to end and form groups of three bases, called *codons* (Figure 1.6). When a codon enters the ribosome, free-floating tRNA molecules consisting of a matching element and an amino acid attempt

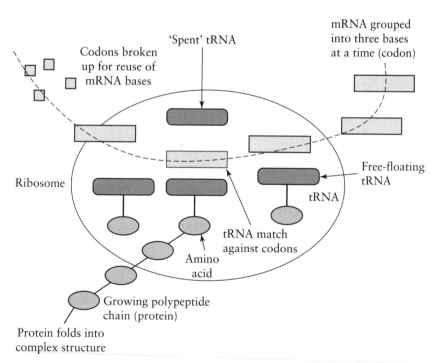

Figure 1.6   The process of translation at a ribosome

to match the codon against their matching element. If a match is made, the attached amino acid is released from the tRNA and added to the amino acid sequence (polypeptide chain) that is being formed from earlier matches against the mRNA that has entered the ribosome. For instance, the mRNA triplet **GCU** (guanine–cytosine–uracil), which is an mRNA transcription of the DNA triplet **CGA** (cytosine–guanine–adenine), is mapped by a tRNA molecule onto the amino acid *alanine*.

The spent mRNA can be reused in the nucleus for the formation of new mRNA. The spent tRNA can be reused if another amino acid is attached to the matching element. At initiation the ribosome recognizes the starting point in a segment of mRNA and binds a molecule of tRNA bearing a single amino acid. In elongation, a second amino acid is linked to the first, the ribosome shifts position on the mRNA molecule, and the elongation cycle is repeated. When a stop codon is reached, the chain of amino acids folds spontaneously to form a protein.

The start of gene translation is signalled by a specific sequence, **AUG** (*methionine*), and translated proteins will nearly always start with M. However, if there is a jump in transcription and a base is skipped over, a shift in the 'reading frame' results, leading to different codons and a different sequence of amino acids for the same sequence of DNA. While such shifts will mostly result from errors in transcription, it is possible that such jumps are also part of normal transcription, resulting in a gene producing up to three different transcripts of a coding region depending on whether it jumps over no bases, one base or two bases at the start of the transcription process.

There are 64 different combinations of mRNA nucleotides in codons: four ways to form the first base times four ways to form the second base times four ways to form the third base. Although there are 64 different codons, there are only 20 amino acids used by the human body and the vast majority of organisms on this planet. The translation of codons into amino acids by 64 different tRNA molecules, each with their own matching element, is determined by the 'genetic code' (Table 1.1). Many scientists believe that the best evidence that all life on Earth evolved from a common ancestor three billion years or so ago comes from the fact that the genetic code is universal for nearly all life on Earth. The amino acid names and commonly accepted ways to abbreviate them are given in Table 1.2. A typical gene sequence and its protein product are given in Table 1.3.

Once the full protein sequence consisting of amino acids linked together by tRNA and synthesized by ribosomes is formed, it goes through

Table 1.1   The mRNA genetic code: 61 mRNA codons stand for one of the 20 amino acids; the remaining three – **ATT, ATC** and **ACT** in DNA form, **UAA, UAG** and **UGA** in mRNA form (above) – are used for 'punctuation' and tell the tRNA to stop translation (i.e. the end of the gene has been reached). Only small variations to this genetic code exist in a few microbes, and the genetic code applies to all nuclear genes, i.e. genes which are enveloped in a nucleus within a cell, as opposed to DNA which is free-floating within the cell. The genetic code can also be expressed in DNA terms (e.g. **TTT** for Phe, etc.).

First base	Second base				Third base
	U	C	A	G	
U	UUU Phe	UCU Ser	UAU Tyr	UGU Cys	U
	UUC Phe	UCC Ser	UAC Tyr	UGC Cys	C
	UUA Leu	UCA Ser	UAA Stop	UGA Stop	A
	UUG Leu	UCG Ser	UAG Stop	UGG Trp	G
C	CUU Leu	CCU Pro	CAU His	CGU Arg	U
	CUC Leu	CCC Pro	CAC His	CGC Arg	C
	CUA Leu	CCA Pro	CAA Gln	CGA Arg	A
	CUG Leu	CCG Pro	CAG Gln	CGG Arg	G
A	AUU Ile	ACU Thr	AAU Asn	AGU Ser	U
	AUC Ile	ACC Thr	AAC Asn	AGC Ser	C
	AUA Ile	ACA Thr	AAA Lys	AGA Arg	A
	AUG Met	ACG Thr	AAG Lys	AGG Arg	G
G	GUU Val	GCU Ala	GAU Asp	GGU Gly	U
	GUC Val	GCC Ala	GAC Asp	GGC Gly	C
	GUA Val	GCA Ala	GAA Glu	GGA Gly	A
	GUG Val	GCG Ala	GAG Glu	GGG Gly	G

a post-translational process whereby it first folds into a complex three-dimensional structure in the Endoplasmic Reticulum and then enters the Golgi apparatus for further modification, such as the addition of sugar molecules and other markers that help the protein find its localization (that is, where in the cell or in other cells it should go). Only after these post-translational modifications is the protein functional. The collection of all proteins produced in a cell, in tissue, organ or organism is called the *proteome*, and the study of proteins is *proteomics*.

Summary of transcription and translation

To summarize, collisions between RNA polymerase (an enzyme which is a large protein that helps make and break bonds) and the DNA lead to the RNA polymerase running into certain initiation and start sequences of genes and latching onto them.

Table 1.2   The 20 amino acids and their commonly used abbreviations; each amino acid has a single letter as well as a three-letter abbreviation (Table 1.1).

Full name	Single-letter abbreviation	Three-letter abbreviation
Glycine	G	GLY Gly
Alanine	A	ALA Ala
Valine	V	VAL Val
Leucine	L	LEU Leu
Isoleucine	I	ILE Ile
Phenylalanine	F	PHE Phe
Proline	P	PRO Pro
Serine	S	SER Ser
Threonine	T	THR Thr
Cysteine	C	CYS Cys
Methionine	M	MET Met
Tryptophan	W	TRP Trp
Tyrosine	T	TYR Tyr
Asparagine	N	ASN Asn
Glutamine	Q	GLN Gln
Aspartic acid	D	ASP Asp
Glutamic acid	E	GLU Glu
Lysine	K	LYS Lys
Arginine	R	ARG Arg
Histidine	H	HIS His

The RNA polymerase then unravels the appropriate part of the DNA double helix. Free-floating bases in the nucleus attach themselves to the revealed DNA bases on the template strand, forming a complementary sequence which becomes the messenger RNA. The double helix is re-formed as transcription continues along the unravelled DNA molecule. When a terminating sequence of bases is found in the DNA, the resulting messenger RNA, after editing to remove introns and to form alternative spliced forms, is dispatched to the ribosomes, where combinations of three bases at a time in the messenger RNA are used by tRNA to produce one of 20 different amino acids. Sequences of these amino acids (varying in length from a few hundred to a few thousand) are called polypeptide chains, which are folded in the Endoplasmic Reticulum and packaged in the Golgi apparatus and then (i) secreted from the cell as enzymes and proteins for use by other cells in the organism, or (ii) used by the cell for its own purposes (as, for example, with single cell organisms). These polypeptide chains are therefore the final representation, or product, of the sequence of bases unravelled in the DNA molecule.

Table 1.3 An example of a gene and its amino acid translation, taken from http://www.ncbi.nlm.nih.gov/entrez. The mRNA sequence is given in (a) and consists of 729 bases. The name of the gene is given by the 'Locus' field in (c), with its definition below. A unique accession number for the gene is also provided (Z22865). The source of the gene is provided in terms of discoverers and authors. The 'CDS' values indicate that only bases 13 to 618 result in translation after editing. Hence, translation starts with the 'aug' sequence at positions 13, 14 and 15 in (a). This codon is mapped to methionine (M) in (b) (see Table 1.1). The next codon 'gac' is translated to aspartic acid (D), and so on. The final codon (positions 616, 617 and 618) is 'uag', which stands for 'stop'. Hence the final translated codon is in positions 613, 614 and 615 (guu), which is valine (V)

(a)

```
  1 gaauucggga gcauggaccu cagucuucuc uggguacuua ugccccuagu caccauggcc
 61 uggggccagu auggcgauua uggauaccca uaccagcagu aucaugacua cagcgaugau
121 ggguggguga auuugaaucg gcaaggcuuc agcuaccagu guccccaggg gcaggugaua
181 guggccguga ggagcaucuu caguaagaag gaagguucug acagacaaug gaacuacgcc
241 ugcaugccca cgccacagag ccucggggaa cccacggagu gcuggguggga ggagaucaac
301 agggcuggca uggaauggua ccagacgugc uccaacaaug ggcuggucggc aggauuccag
361 agccgcuacu ucgagucagu gcuggaucgg gaguggcagu uuuacuguug ucgcuacagc
421 aagaggugcc cauauuccug cuggcuaaca acagaauauc caggucacua uggugaggaa
481 auggacauga uuuccuacaa uuaugauuac uauauccgag gagcaacaac cacuuucucu
541 gcaguggaaa gggaucgcca guggaaguuc auaaugugcc ggaugacuga auacgacugu
601 gaauuugcaa auguuuagau uugccacaua ccaaaucugg gugaaaggaa aggggcccuc
661 cagcuuucca cugcagagaa agugguuguu gcuccucggu auauguaaac auaauuguag
721 aucgaauuc
```

(b)

MDLSLLWVLMPLVTMAWGQYGDYGYPYQQYHDYSDDGWVNLNRQGFSY
QCPQGQVIVAVRSIFSKKEGSDRQWNYACMPTPQSLGEPTECWWEEINRAGM
EWYQTCSNNGLVAGFQSRYFESVLDREWQFYCCRYSKRCPYSCWLTTEYPGH
YGEEMDMISYNYDYYIRGATTTFSAVERDRQWKFIMCRMTEYDCEFANV

(c)

LOCUS	HSDERMATA	729 bp
DEFINITION	H.sapiens dermatopontin mRNA, complete CDS	
ACCESSION	Z22865	
KEYWORDS	dermatopontin; proteoglycan-binding cell-adhesion protein	
REFERENCE	1 (bases 1 to 729)	
AUTHORS	Superti-Furga, A., Rocchi, M., Schafer, B.W. and Gitzelmann, R.	
TITLE	Complementary DNA sequence and chromosomal mapping of a human proteoglycan-binding cell-adhesion protein (dermatopontin)	
JOURNAL	*Genomics* **17** (2), 463–467 (1993)	
CDS	13....618	

1.5 Current knowledge and the 'central dogma'

What has been described so far is the 'central dogma' in biology: that one gene by and large produces one mRNA that by and large produces one protein. More specifically, the central dogma consists of six 'axioms'.

1 DNA replicates its information in a process that involves many replication enzymes.

2 DNA codes for the production of messenger RNA (mRNA) during transcription.

3 In eukaryotic cells, the mRNA is processed (essentially by splicing) and migrates from the nucleus to the cytoplasm.

4 mRNA carries coded information to ribosomes, where protein is synthesized using the mRNA during translation.

5 Proteins do not code for the production of proteins, RNA or DNA.

6 Proteins are involved in almost all biological activities, structural or enzymatic.

In fact, transcription and translation are even more complicated than previously described. Some gene products are not translated at all but function in their RNA form after transcription. For instance, genes that code for tRNA and ribosomes cannot be translated. If they could, they would depend on tRNA and ribosomes for the translation! Instead, after transcription these RNA molecules exit the nucleus and perform their roles in the translation of normally transcribed and translated genes. This has led to the identification of several different types of RNA, the most common of which are messenger RNA (mRNA), transfer RNA (tRNA), ribosomal RNA (rRNA) for the building of the ribosomes, and small nuclear RNA (snRNA) that help edit the mRNA. mRNA is the primary messenger synthesized from a gene segment of DNA and carrying the code into the cytoplasm where protein synthesis occurs. rRNA (ribosomal) in the cytoplasm and protein combine to form a nucleoprotein (ribosome) that serves as the translation site and carries the enzymes necessary for protein synthesis. Several ribosomes may be attached to a single mRNA at any time. tRNA (transfer) contains about 75 nucleotides, three of which form a tRNA anticodon, and one amino acid. The tRNA reads the code and carries the amino acid to be incorporated into the developing protein.

Also, there is growing evidence that, for many genes, there are many more 'splice variants' than previously believed, where different combinations of introns and exons exist. It is not a simple matter of introns being removed and the remaining exons being sent sequentially to the ribosomes. One gene can produce many different types of polypeptide chain depending on how many introns are removed and how the exons are shuffled or differently spliced. This means that, while the human genome may consist of only 30 000 genes, the genes may produce many more proteins. It is not currently clear what the relationship between gene and protein is in humans, or how many human genes can be alternatively spliced, but estimates vary from between 1:10 to 1:100 for the gene: protein ratio and from 60 per cent up to 75 per cent of human genes having alternative splice variants. That is, although humans have only 30 000 genes, these may well produce anything between 200 000 and two million proteins through alternative splicing. Interest in splice variants has led to the conjecture that, in addition to the genome (total set of DNA and genes) and proteome (total set of proteins), it is in the spliceosome (total set of alternative splice variants for a particular gene) that the real answers will be found as to how genes are mapped onto proteins and how many proteins are actually capable of being made.

DNA polymerase which replicates chromosomes is so accurate that there is only one error in every 10^7 nucleotide pairs. A DNA mismatch repair system also operates to correct nearly all of these errors, increasing the overall accuracy to one error in 10^9 nucleotides copied. While thousands of random chemical changes are created every day in human DNA, the vast majority are eliminated by DNA repair. For instance, some varieties of yeast have about 50 genes devoted to gene repair. It is not known how many human genes are devoted to gene repair.

The Mendelian concept of dominant and recessive genes can be given precise biomolecular accounts in terms of genes which express their effects via proteins even in the presence of a different gene for the same trait ('dominant') and genes which do not produce an observable effect via proteins when paired with a dominant gene ('recessive'). When a new diploid cell is formed, complete copies of all the chromosomes must be made through DNA replication. The two copies of a chromosome pair have the same genes but may have different versions (alleles) of these genes with distinct DNA sequences. So, for instance, if there is a single gene for the colour of hair, it will have many forms, each coding for a certain hair colour. There will be two such genes – one inherited from the father and the other from the mother. One may be dominant and the other recessive, in which case hair will be produced of similar colour to one of the parents, or both could be dominant or recessive, in which case hair will be produced that is the 'average' between the parents' hair colour. It is also possible that one allele could be dominant for a certain period, and then be suppressed by the other allele for other periods.

1.6 Why proteins are important

So, what happens to the enzymes/proteins produced by ribosomes, the Endoplasmic Reticulum and the Golgi apparatus? As mentioned earlier, proteins carry out many vital functions in living organisms. As structural molecules, they provide much of the cytoskeletal framework of cells and also help cells form tissue. Proteins also carry signals from one part of the body to another, or from one cell to another. Proteins can also act as a transport system, carrying molecules such as oxygen in the circulatory system so that all cells can have access to this important element. The human immune system is also dependent on proteins for detecting the arrival of pathogens as they enter the human system and for helping to mount an effective immune system defence. As *enzymes* proteins act as biological catalysts that speed up the rate of cellular reactions. The chemical composition of one cell could be placed in a test tube and observed. After some time, some chemical reactions naturally occurring in the test tube might be noted. There will be a long delay because the activation energy required to start a chemical reaction acts like an energy barrier over which the molecules must be raised for a reaction to take place. An enzyme effectively lowers the activation energy required for a reaction to proceed. An enzyme locks onto a molecule, starts a reaction, and then is released unchanged. The rate of enzyme combination and release is called the *turnover rate* and is about 1000 times a second for most enzymes, with variation between 100 per s and 10 million per s. The increase in reaction rate achieved by enzymes ranges from a minimum of about a million to as much as a trillion times faster than an uncatalysed reaction at equivalent concentrations and temperatures.

However, enzymes cannot work unless they have folded in the right way. That is, it is the structure of the enzyme that determines what it does and whether it does it. If enzymes do not fold in the right way, they cannot carry out their enzymatic activity, because they will not be able to lock on to their target molecules (which also have complex three-dimensional structures) to start the appropriate reaction. The study of protein folding and protein structure is a key element in understanding what proteins do. However, what is actually observed in organisms are already-folded proteins. Trying to 'straighten' a protein so that the sequence of amino acids is revealed is a major problem in proteomics. The number of well-understood, sequenced and structured proteins is small compared with the total number of proteins that exist. Also, as will be seen later, trying to determine the structure of a protein from its DNA, mRNA or even amino acid sequence is much more complex than it appears. There is therefore a growing mismatch between understanding genes and mRNA (which is growing rapidly) and their resulting proteins (which is growing much more slowly). However, genes and mRNA do not carry out the crucial work required in a cell or organism – proteins do. A key question for bioinformatics is whether this growing gap between knowledge of genes and knowledge of proteins can somehow be bridged by the use of computers.

From this it can be seen that the process of enzyme/protein production, as determined by DNA, is absolutely critical to the continued well-being of an organism, otherwise organisms as chemical beings would not produce chemical reactions fast enough to keep then alive (e.g. respiration, digestion). Enzymes degrade eventually after catalysing many reactions, and they are broken down into their constituent parts by other enzymes (the 'degradome') for reuse by the organism.

What life now means, according to biomolecular science, is the set of genes (DNA) which code for the production of appropriate enzymes which increase the rate of chemical reactions in cells, where the nature and rate of reactions are determined by the nature of the enzymes. Organisms of a particular species are all essentially the same chemically; what differs are the enzymes produced by the DNA inherited by their parents and other factors (e.g. mutation of individual bases and genes by random means). These enzymes control cellular processes differently for different members of the species, thereby leading to different physical characteristics.

1.7 Gene and cell regulation

It is necessary to assume that there is some 'control' mechanism that regulates gene transcription (into mRNA) and mRNA translation (into polypeptide chains). If transcription and translation were only dependent on random collisions thousands, if not millions, of times per s deep within the nucleus (transcription) and at ribosomes (translation), there would be no cell differentiation, since each cell would transcribe and translate its full complement of DNA. Yet, there are many different types of cell producing different types of protein from different subsets of their genes. Cells of the same type form tissue, and tissues form organs, resulting in an organism where it is the differences in cell type which give the organism its shape and structure. If all cells transcribed their full complement of DNA, organisms would be shapeless and lack structure.

Transcriptional regulation helps to determine which parts of a genome are active in a nucleus (i.e. can be copied into mRNA) and which are de-activated. Translational regulation determines the rate at which mRNAs copied from active genes are used by ribosomes in protein synthesis. Genes coding for mRNA are much longer than their corresponding mRNA, consisting of a flanking region upstream of the first nucleotide to be copied. This flanking region consists of a *promoter* and an *enhancer*. The promoter itself consists of two parts: *basal* and *upstream*. The basal promoter provides recognition and binding sites for the RNA polymerase II (pol II, or RNAP II) and is located about 40 base pairs (bps) from the start of the gene. The basal promoter attracts a large number of other proteins to it called *transcription factors*, the function of which is to initiate accurate transcription of the gene. The basal promoter typically contains a sequence of seven bases (**TATAAAA**, the 'TATA box' see Figure 1.4). Upstream promoters serve to activate or repress transcription, and once the basal promoter is occupied, several other proteins attach themselves to the basal promoter or upstream stretches of DNA to modulate the rate of transcription, including repressing the gene altogether.

Although the precise details are not yet fully understood, it appears that promoters and enhancers form a DNA sequence, called a *cis* element, which is recognized by a regulatory protein, called a *trans* element. Several genes may have the same *cis* element which is recognized by the same *trans* element, which can both increase and decrease the rate of initiation, typically a thousandfold. Many eukaryotic genes are controlled in groups or networks, whereby a *trans* element (regulatory protein) increases or decreases the rate of initiation of a number of genes, one or more of which in turn code for other *trans* elements (regulatory proteins) which control the rate of initiation of still other genes.

Regulatory proteins are themselves the result of prior transcription and translation of other parts of the DNA. Interestingly, if each gene had its own unique *cis* element, then there would be as many *trans* elements as genes. The question of where these *trans* elements come from would in turn require still other genes, which require their own *trans* elements, ad infinitum. This still leaves the question of where the first *trans* element comes from. One approach is to focus on the ability of a gene, because of its biomolecular structure and content, to *self-transcribe* without the need for transcription mechanisms such as polymerase and promoters. Another approach is to hypothesize that, at the moment of fertilization, the cell contains not just genetic information but also some basic transcription mechanisms and other elements (perhaps in the nucleolus – a subpart of the nucleus) to bootstrap the process of transcription and translation.

1.8 When cell regulation goes wrong

In addition to gene regulation, there is also cell regulation. Cells are programmed to divide and make copies of themselves at certain times, depending on the type of cell. The process of *mitotic cell division* consists of several phases, including chromosome replication and the division of the cell into two daughter cells. For instance, skin cells, white blood cells and stomach cells have to be replaced frequently (every few days), whereas nerve cells and muscle cells have much longer lifespans. It is estimated that normal cells can divide between 40 and 70 times. The limit for cell division is reached when the chromosomes in a cell, which are 'shortened' each time they replicate, are too short for further replication. This shortening occurs because the molecules responsible for chromosome replication start a little way in from the ends of chromosomes (*telomeres*) for each replication. At some stage the telomeres no longer protect the DNA on chromosomes, and replication is no longer possible without the formation of incomplete chromosomes. Malformed daughter cells then result which can no longer function as replacements. Normal cell division is also required for growth from child to mature adult, and repair if tissue is damaged. The human body experiences a constant turnover of cells as some die and others reproduce and replace them. However, the process of orderly reproduction of cells can go wrong, and this can lead to one of over 100 diseases generically called *cancer*.

The current model of cancer is as follows. DNA in cells can be mutated as a result of exposure to the environment (e.g. radiation), *carcinogens* (biological or chemical substances that are believed to cause cancer) and some *pathogens* (Hepatitus B and C viruses cause a significant number of liver cancers). Mostly such mutations are in non-coding sections of a cell's DNA or genes that do not affect cell replication. However, sometimes these mutations affect genes that are critical for the timing of cell division (*proto-oncogenes*), which then become oncogenes that instruct a cell to divide repeatedly without control. Usually, the cell has other genes for countering such mutations, but if these other genes are also affected then the cell forms a *tumour* (a mass of cells) that continues to grow. Somehow cancer cells achieve 'immortality' in that telomere reduction with each replication does not appear to affect the ability of the tumour to grow. Many tumours are *benign* or non-malignant in that they do not pose a danger, as long as there is room for growth of the tumour; but if the tumour blocks the normal functioning of other cells, or if the tumour *metastatizes* (cancerous cells can move from part of the body to another if they enter the circulatory system) and starts developing in other parts of the body so that they become life-threatening, the tumour becomes *malignant*. For instance, melanoma is a cancer of pigmented skin cells which is usually benign, but if melanoma cells enter the bloodstream they can be transported to the liver and brain, where they can present a real danger by blocking the development of normal cells in surrounding tissue.

1.9 So, what is bioinformatics?

There are many ways in which computer science can help in molecular biology research. Here are just a few, to give an idea of how computers can be useful in biology.

1 The use of computer technology for storing DNA sequence information and constructing the correct DNA sequences from fragments identified by restriction enzymes (enzymes which break up the DNA at certain points) was one of the first applications, arising from the Human Genome Project and other projects dealing with sequencing the DNA of various organisms. While the DNA in a set of 23 chromosomes for a human is about 3.5 Gigabytes, the *H. influenzae* genome is only 1.9 Mbs, *E. coli* about 4.6 Mbs, and *C.elegans* about 97 Mbs. Various projects are already underway to sequence the genomes of chicken and buffalo, and these projects, as well as several others, will lead to huge data storage and access requirements.

2 Once genome sequences are stored and accessed, there is a need for comparative genome analysis across databases so that the organization and evolution of genomes can be studied. Such analyses may

uncover relationships between model organisms, crops, domestic animals and humans. Visualization tools and techniques are required to
conduct these analyses.

3   Large databases need to be structured and organized using a common
'ontology', or set of terms which are related structurally to each other,
so that researchers can access data from different databases using the
same 'query language'. The *Gene Ontology Consortium* has produced
controlled vocabularies for describing genes and proteins which, it is
hoped, will be used by all bioinformaticians so that a common way
of referring to genes and their products emerges.

4   Many areas of biology rely on images for communicating their results. Tools and techniques are required for searching, describing,
manipulating and analysing for features within these images.

5   Once databases of genomes are created, there is a need for maintaining these databases and for checking that their contents are error-free
and valid as researchers add new information. Anomalies must be
identified and actions taken to ensure that the databases are as con-
sistent as possible.

6   Protein sequences are being added to protein databases, and while
these are not growing as quickly as genomic databases, there is
a need to store protein sequences and their structure as well as
their function. Even if a common vocabulary for describing proteins is accepted, there is a major need to link protein sequences
with their DNA source sequences, given the problems of introns
and non-coding DNA. There is also a need for tools that can predict the structure of a protein from its sequence of amino acids
(Chapter 2).

1.10 Summary of chapter

1   Genes in DNA are made up of sequences of four bases and are transcribed into messenger RNA transcripts. It is currently not known
how many transcripts can be formed from each human gene, and
therefore it is currently not known how many products there are for
any specific human gene.

2 One gene on one strand of the double-helix (the template) is used to make the transcript. Genes are transcribed from the 3' to 5' end, and so the mRNA is synthesized from the 5' to 3' end.

3 mRNA is complementary to the source or template strand, except that T in DNA is replaced by U in the mRNA. When DNA replicates to make a complete copy of itself for cell division, normal complementary base copying occurs.

4 Genes code not only for structural and enzymatic proteins but also for products that can affect the rate at which genes are transcribed. Various transcription factors determine which genes are transcribed in a particular cell.

5 Various transcription factors bind to upstream promoter regions of genes and regulate the rate of transcription and whether a gene should be transcribed.

6 mRNA transcripts are themselves edited to form alternative splice variants, whereby exons coding for proteins survive and introns that are not meant for translation to protein are removed.

1.11 Further reading

Griffiths, A.J.F., Miller, J.H., Suzuki, D.T., *et al.* (2005) *Introduction to Genetic Analysis*, 8th edn, Freeman.

Latchman, D. (1995) *Gene Regulation*, Stanley Thornes.

Mount, D.W. (2001) *Bioinformatics: Sequence and Genome Analysis*, Cold Spring Harbor Laboratory Press.

Weaver, R.F. (2002) *Molecular Biology*, McGraw Hill.

2

Introduction to Problems and Challenges in Bioinformatics

2.1 Introduction

Chapter 1 provided an overview of the basics of molecular biology of relevance to bioinformaticians and also introduced some of the initial problems faced by researchers in the area. This chapter examines current and future challenges in bioinformatics. The problem areas and challenges are presented according to the field of molecular biology in which they occur: the genome, the transcriptome and the proteome. Also, the recently expanding area of gene silencing and interference technology will be covered.

2.2 Genome

Sequence analysis

Some of the earliest problems in genomics concerned how to measure similarity of DNA and protein sequences, either within a genome, or across the genomes of different individuals, or across the genomes of different species. DNA and proteins can be similar in terms of their *function*, their *structure* or their linear sequence of nucleotides or amino acids. The fundamental assumption for DNA is that two DNA sequences that are similar probably share the same function, even if they occur in different parts of the genome or across two or more genomes. The fundamental

Intelligent Bioinformatics   Edward Keedwell and Ajit Narayanan
© 2005 John Wiley & Sons, Ltd

assumption for proteins is that linear sequence determines *shape* which, in turn, determines function. This is because the shape of a protein, and in particular of enzymes, determines which other molecules these proteins can lock on to and affect.

Consider the two DNA strings of equal length: **ACGTACGT** and **AC-CTAGGT**. How similar are they? One way to deal with this problem is to place them one on top of the other:

A	C	G	T	A	C	G	T
A	C	C	T	A	G	G	T

A count is made column by column to identify the number of mismatches per position, which in the above case is two. This is the *Hamming distance*, which is the simplest measure of similarity available. The two strings **ACGTACGT** and **CCCTCCCT** would have a Hamming distance of four, and the two strings **ACCTAGGT** and **CCCTCCCT** would also have a Hamming distance of four. The two strings **ACGTACGT** and **AC-CTAGGT** therefore are more similar to each other (Hamming distance of two) than **CCCTCCCT** is to either of them (Hamming distance of four). The problem is, what happens if strings are of unequal length? Consider **ACGTACGT** and **AGTACGT**. If these strands are lined up:

A	C	G	T	A	C	G	T
A	G	T	A	C	G	T	

the result is a Hamming distance of seven (assuming that the last base of the first string cannot be matched to a blank). Yet, if a blank is inserted in the second string:

A	C	G	T	A	C	G	T
A	-	G	T	A	C	G	T

the Hamming distance is one, i.e. the strings are very similar.

Now imagine that, instead of just eight bases in a DNA sequence there are hundreds and possibly thousands of bases (for example, if a whole gene is compared against other genes). Gene sequences are extremely unlikely to be of equal length, and methods must be found for inserting blanks at appropriate locations in the shorter string and stretching it out to optimize the number of matches. Shorter strings may result when the DNA replication machinery goes wrong and bases are skipped over.

Equally, some bases may need to be deleted. Consider the following three strings:

A	C	G	T	A	C	G	T
A	G	T	A	C	G	T	
A	G	G	A	C	G	T	

One possibility is to insert blanks into the second and third strings at position two (two insertions) to line up the three strings. Another possibility is to delete the second base of the first string (one deletion):

A	G	T	A	C	G	T
A	G	T	A	C	G	T
A	G	G	A	C	G	T

Since one deletion may be preferable to two insertions this may be the preferred strategy, but now consider what would happen if the first two strings were matched without any knowledge of the third string. The strategy might well have been to insert a blank into position two of the second string to optimize similarity. However, when the third string is entered, it is now discovered that it would have been preferable to delete the second base of the first string rather than insert a blank into the third string. Backtracking may be required to undo the insertion of the blank into the second string, but backtracking will only work if there is stored information as to what was done earlier so that it can be undone. For long strings and for matching many strings, the memory requirements can quickly become large.

The above problem is easy with just a handful of strings and small numbers of bases, but already the problem with long and large numbers of sequences is apparent. There can be *pairwise comparison* of strings, where changes are made to earlier decisions as new strings are entered, or there can be *multiple comparison* of all strings at once and matches can be optimized for specific positions across all sequences. Also, there can be *local alignment* (finding alignments between parts of two or more sequences) and *global alignment* (finding an alignment for sequences in their entirety). There are now a number of publicly available tools on the web for undertaking alignments.[1,2]

The requirement for a minimal number of changes arises from the principle that, when identifying similarity between strings, as few alterations

---

[1] See, for example, http://www.ncbi.nlm.nih.gov/Education/ for a tutorial on Blast.
[2] See, for example, http://www.ebi.ac.uk/fasta33 for Fasta.

as possible should be made to the original strings so that optimal similarity measures are returned. This is the *unit cost* model, also known as the Levenshtein Distance, which states that the cost of an alignment of two sequences s_1 and s_2 is the sum of the costs of all the 'edit' operations required to match the two sequences, and that an *optimal* alignment of s_1 and s_2 is an alignment that has minimal cost among all the possible ways that they can be aligned. Extensions to the unit cost model include *substitution matrices* that provide variable costs for insertion, deletion and replacement of bases and amino acids, *realistic gap models* that prevent deletions and insertions in critical subsequences (such as strongly conserved subunits in protein sequences involved in protein–protein interaction, where any edit in these subsequences may destroy the desired biochemical function) and the use of an extended genetic alphabet that represents possible ambiguities in the data. The most common symbols used in an extended genetic alphabet are: **R** for **G** or **A** (PuRine), **Y** for **T** or **C** (PYramidine) and **N** (ANy).

A related problem here is how to find a common substring for all strings or sequences. This is known as the 'superstring' problem, where the common substring is the shortest sequence of characters shared by all sequences. This problem is, in computational terms, *intractable*, in that there is no known algorithm that will work in reasonable time to find such a superstring as the number of sequences and their length increase.

Phylogeny

Many algorithms now exist for sequence alignment, including Dynamic Programming (for both pairwise and multiple alignment) and the Carillo–Lipman method for optimal multiple alignment. The purpose of alignment is to learn about the phylogenetic and evolutionary relationships between genes with a similar function. For instance, a large number of sequences can be retrieved from a number of different genome or protein databases using a specific subsequence. Each database may store information on one or more organisms. The research task is then to discover the evolutionary relationships between these sequences and therefore the organisms on the assumption that evolution can be described as 'descent with modification'. That is, inherited similarities and differences between organisms provide the basic information needed to hypothesize evolutionary relationships between these organisms, where these similarities and differences are expressed in DNA sequences, amino acid sequences or phenotypic characteristics. The principle of *parsimony* in phylogeny essentially states that derived similarities between sequences can be assumed to be caused by common ancestry and that inferences concerning these similarities should be kept as simple as possible.

Phylogeny and classification are important areas of biology, since they deal with the identification, naming and grouping of organisms based on shared similarities. Linnaeus introduced the 'binomial' classification system in the 18th century consisting of two Latin names, where the first name (always starting with a capital letter) denotes the *genus* and the second (always starting with a lower case) the *species* (as in *Homo sapiens*). While only two layers of taxonomy existed in Linnaeus' day, it is currently widely accepted that there are seven layers: *Kingdom, Phylum, Class, Order, Family, Genus, species*. The task of current phylogeny is to locate all organisms in a comprehensive classification scheme that reflects their evolution from a common ancestor believed to have come into existence about two and a half to three billion years ago on this planet.

To give an idea of the computational cost involved in such a comprehensive classification, imagine that all organisms have just five genes, each of which can take any number of alleles. Gene sequences can be compared base by base, as previously described, to identify similarities and differences between genes. Imagine also initially that there are just four organisms, each of which takes 1 s to compare with another organism across all five genes. To construct a set of similarity scores for these four organisms takes 6 s (3 s to compare organism 1 with organisms 2, 3 and 4; 2 s to compare organism 2 with 3 and 4; and 1 s to compare organism 3 with 4). If there are 10 organisms, the time taken is 9 + 8 + ... 1 = 45 s. That is, to calculate similarity scores for n organisms takes $(n-1)*(n/2)$ s. The cost for 100 organisms is therefore 99*50 s = 4950 s, or 1 h 22.5 min. Note that the time taken for 100 organisms is not the same as 25 times the cost for four organisms. It is estimated that there are between 12 and 15 million existing organisms/species on this planet, with some claims that 99 per cent of species are extinct. To calculate similarity scores for 10 million existing species, given previous assumptions, would take 9 999 999*5 000 000 s, i.e. over one and a half million years. If this represents just 1 per cent of all species, it will take us over 150 million years to calculate similarities for all organisms that have ever existed. If it is argued that 1 s per comparison is far too long, given just four genes, it can be counter-argued that organisms contain more than just four genes, so even this figure will need amending upwards. Even if it is possible to calculate the similarities in a realistic amount of time, there is another problem which is the construction of the resulting

Table 2.1   A table of information indicating shared gene 'values' across four organisms. The gene values are assumed to be binary phenotypic values for the sake of exposition although in real life gene values can be expected to be much more complex, such as long strings of DNA, amino acids or multivalued phenotypes. '0' stands for 'ground state' and '1' for 'advanced state'.

	Gene 1	Gene 2	Gene 3	Gene 4
Organism A	0	0	0	0
Organism B	1	0	0	0
Organism C	1	1	0	1
Organism D	1	0	1	1

phylogenetic tree (a tree diagram that displays evolutionary relationships among a number of organisms or species).

Consider Table 2.1 and the four organisms with the four genes that they share. For the sake of simplicity, assume that each gene has only two phenotypic values, 0 and 1. The task here, however, is to demonstrate the complexity involved in generating phylogenetic trees for even this simple dataset.

The values for genes differ between different organisms through a variety of mechanisms. Mutations (that is, value differences) can occur through substitution (one nucleotide miscopied as another), insertions (new bases are added) and deletions (some bases are deleted altogether), resulting in different gene values, as in Table 2.1. The question arises as to whether, given the information in Table 2.1, any overall conclusions can be drawn as to how these organisms are related in evolutionary terms to each other.

There are two general methods for deriving trees from such tables. The first, called *Hennig Argumentation*, considers the information provided by each gene one at a time (i.e. it works column by column). The information in Gene 1 (advanced state value 1) unites B, C and D (Figure 2.1(a)), the information in Gene 2 (advanced state value 1) is peculear to C (Figure 2.1(b)), the information in Gene 3 (advanced state value 1) is peculear to D (Figure 2.1(c)), and finally the information in Gene 4 (advanced state 1) is shared between C and D (Figure 2.1(d)). A tree is obtained that evolves as the information is included column by column.

One interpretation of the tree is that all four organisms shared an ancestor in the past (first split in the tree), but that B, C and D split from A through the sharing of a specific value for Gene 1 (common ancestor for B, C and D), that C and D split from B through the sharing of a

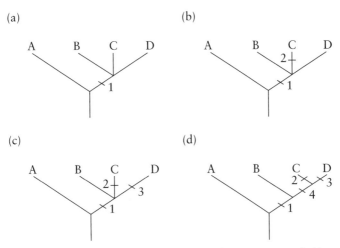

Figure 2.1   Hennig Argumentation considers the information provided by each gene one at a time

specific value for Gene 4 (common ancestor for C and D), and that C and D split from each other through the acquisition of specific values for Genes 2 and 3 (common ancestor).

Hennig Argumentation is simple but can lead to complex tree labelling when information from genes in subsequent columns conflicts with information already included from earlier columns. This can in turn lead to complex interpretations of phylogeny. For instance, if Gene 4 had united B and C rather than C and D, the label for Gene 4 would need to be moved to the same location as the label for Gene 1, and then explicitly an exception label must be inserted to signify that D does not share the value for Gene 4 (Figure 2.2). The interpretation now is that D reverted back to its original state with regard to Gene 4 after a common ancestor to B, C and D shared a common state for Gene 4.

Trees derived through Hennig Argumentation are therefore highly dependent on the first columns (genes) encountered and do not take the information in all columns into account before generating the first candidate phylogeny tree. Conflicts in subsequent columns can lead to many exception labels or even re-formatting the tree to minimize such exceptions. While the situation may not be too bad for a 'binary' gene value example, real gene values can be expected to consist of more than just binary states, and typically many more than four organisms will need to be related phylogenetically.

To overcome the problems of Hennig Argumentation, *Wagner Trees* can be used instead. Consider the information in Table 2.2, but this time a phylogenetic tree is going to be constructed organism by organism

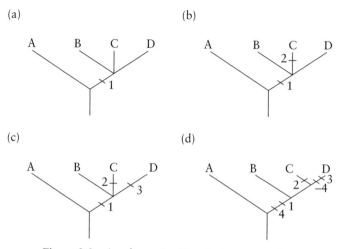

Figure 2.2   An alternative Hennig Argumentation

(row by row) rather than gene by gene (column by column), with the purpose of minimizing the number of state changes required. The first step in Wagner Tree construction is to find the organism that has fewest 'advanced' states, where 1 stands for 'advanced'. A has 0 values across all genes and therefore no advanced states.

A comparison is made between all the other organisms against A, with B having one derived or advanced state in comparison to A, while C and D have two and three derived or advanced states in comparison to A, respectively. B is linked to A first (Figure 2.3(a)) since it is most similar to A. The organism with the next lowest number of advanced states is then identified. Since C has two derived state differences, its name is written beside B and connected to the line that joins B and A (Figure 2.3(b)). At the point where the two lines intersect, the most advanced states present in B and C are listed (the intersection of state values is called an *optimization*). Since B and C both have a derived state for Gene 1 but do not share other derived states, the optimization is 1000, where the first

Table 2.2   A table of gene values for four organisms to demonstrate the Wagner method of phylogenetic tree construction

	Gene 1	Gene 2	Gene 3	Gene 4
Organism A	0	0	0	0
Organism B	1	0	0	0
Organism C	1	1	0	0
Organism D	1	1	1	0

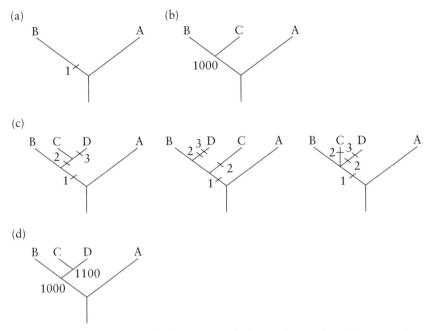

Figure 2.3   The Wagner method constructs phylogenetic trees by adding organisms one at a time based on the number of gene value differences between organisms

bit signifies Gene 1, the second bit Gene 2, and so on. Finally, D has to be linked into the tree and connected to a point that requires the fewest number of state changes. There are several possibilities, three of which are depicted in Figure 2.3 (c). Since the second and third possibilities imply that Gene 2 evolved twice, whereas the first possibility implies that Gene 2 evolved only once, the preferred most *parsimonious* tree (the first possibility) is adopted. An optimization is calculated and the analysis is complete (Figure 2.3 (d)).

To aid tree construction, an *outgroup* organism is usually used that has no shared characteristics (gene values) with any of the organisms to be classified but is nevertheless ancestrally related to the *ingroup* (the organisms to be classified). This outgroup is located in the tree first and acts as a basis for comparison as well as providing 'directionality' to the evolutionary sequence depicted by the tree. The *length* of a tree is the total number of steps or state changes in the tree, and a tree with a smaller length is to be preferred to a tree of greater length for the same organisms. Parsimony is essentially an optimality criterion, and several different methods now exist for calculating optimal tree structures, including Wagner optimality, Fitch optimality, Dollo optimality and Camin–Sokal optimality. Building phylogenetic trees becomes complicated as datasets become larger or contain conflicts that have to be resolved, usually by re-formatting a tree. Optimality procedures usually work in a step-wise manner such that each organism is added where it optimally fits a tree, as in the Wagner method above. However, such *exhaustive* search methods that check all possible trees quickly become intractable as the number of organisms and genes grows.

The ultimate aim of phylogenetic analysis is to present a complete evolutionary history of all life on earth that shows how all organisms are related to each other, either existing or extinct. Advances in molecular biology have now allowed the use of genetic sequences (DNA or amino acid sequences) for tree construction, rather than the characteristic traits that were used in the past, since these sequences provide a more detailed and lower-level account of differences between organisms and species. In Figure 2.4, the top table describes the same stretch of DNA for the four organisms A, B, C and D. B, C and D differ from A in 3, 4 and 5 positions, respectively. B is joined first to A (Figure 2.4(a)) and the optimization is located where their lines join. The three differences between B and A are also described in the order in which the differences appear, working away from where the lines join. C is added next (Figure 2.4(b)) and again the three changes from B are described and the optimization provided. Only two possibilities for joining D are shown here in Figure 2.4(c). Since joining D to C requires fewer changes, this is the chosen tree (Figure 2.4(d)).

2.3 Transcriptome

As previously described in Chapter 1, the total collection of mRNA and their alternative splice forms represents the transcriptome of a cell or organism. The transcriptome can be considered the complete set of instructions for deriving all the different proteins found in a cell or organism. By analysing the transcriptome, it may be possible to discover new proteins that are present in specific tissues or produced only by certain cells under certain conditions. If the genome provides us with the complete set of genes of a cell or organism, and the proteome tells us all of the proteins that can be produced by the genome, the transcriptome is the bridge between the two. If there are more proteins than genes, something must be happening between the genome and proteome to make this possible. By measuring the transcriptome during certain cell development stages, it is possible to identify which genes are switched on or are switched off

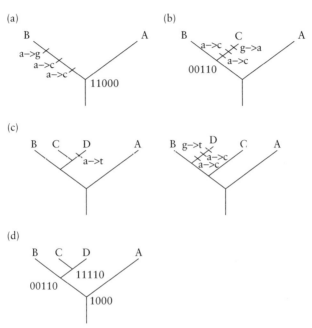

A	a	a	a	a	a
B	a	a	c	c	g
C	c	c	c	c	a
D	c	c	c	c	t

(a)

(b)

(c)

(d)

Figure 2.4 Constructing a phylogenetic tree from example DNA sequences for four organisms A, B, C and D, using the Wagner method

at various points during the process. Also, if the transcriptome can be measured during the development of stem cells, it may also be possible to identify exactly how and when genes are switched on and off so that the cells specialize to become one of the 200 or so different types of cell found in the human body. Such measurement will help answer one of the most profound mysteries in molecular biology, since there is no 'central control' of stem cell division that specializes cells. Specialization of cells must therefore be through some form of signalling pathway through genes.

Interest in the transcriptome (the total set of transcripts possible from the genome, including alternative splice variants) has grown significantly since the arrival of a new technology that allows us to measure both the amount and nature of these transcripts. *DNA arrays* are devices that contain DNA probes that allow complementary mRNA or complementary DNA (cDNA) samples to be bound to the probes. Assume for the moment that the probes are short fragments of each gene that can be found in the genome of an organism, and that the mRNA or cDNA samples are taken from cells or tissues of that same organism under some condition. If the samples are applied to the DNA array and 'stick' to some probes but not others through complementary base pairing, that tells us which genes are expressed in the sample and which genes are not expressed in the sample (Figure 2.5).

The total mRNA from an individual (cell or tissue) is extracted and purified. Since mRNA does not remain stable for long, cDNA versions of the mRNA are reverse transcribed so that the mRNA and cDNA form a stable structure. The strands are then further amplified or transcribed to generate further cDNA or mRNA (called cRNA) strands before being 'labelled'. Typically, samples from one cell or individual are labelled green and samples from another cell or individual red to allow for differential comparison between the samples. The samples are then fragmented into smaller substrands, and the gene chip/microarray is applied. The gene chip/microarray will contain probe nucleotide sequences that uniquely

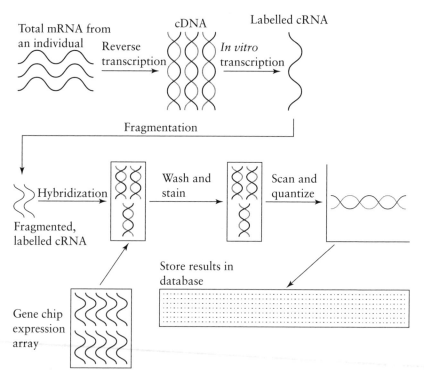

Figure 2.5   Microarray and gene chip measurement (see http://www.affymetrix.com)

detect the presence of its cDNA or mRNA counterpart, if it is present in the sample. The samples are washed over the gene chip/microarray and allowed to 'hybridize' (form short complementary base pairings) with the probes. The gene chip/microarray is then 'read' with a laser that is tuned to measure probes hybridized with green or red samples. If both samples contain equal amounts of the same mRNA/cDNA, the probe will fluoresce an orange/yellow colour. If one of the samples contains more of one form of mRNA/cDNA than another, it will fluoresce either green or red, depending on which sample it came from. If there are no mRNA/cDNA samples for a particular probe, the probe will reflect black or the background colour of the gene chip/microarray. Because the laser reads probes at a certain frequency, the intensity of reflected light can be converted into measures of amount of mRNA/cDNA and stored in a database for further analysis.

There are two main types of DNA array: *microarray* and *DNA* or *gene chip*, depending on how probes (nucleotide sequences) are put onto the chip. Microarrays use presynthesized DNA (about 100 bases) for probing, whereas DNA chips use *in situ* synthesized oligonucleotide probes (25 bases for Affymetrix gene chips). More recently, types of array are distinguished by the amount of genes that can be measured, since DNA chips allow for increased numbers of probes due to their shorter length (between 30 000 and 4 million probes for DNA chips, as opposed to about 20 000 probes for microarrays). Microarrays generally use *spot* technology, whereby a robot places spots (roughly 0.1 μm to 0.5 μm) of DNA on a glass slide (the microarray) and each spot is a DNA counterpart to one of the mRNAs to be measured. These DNA spots act as probes and are generally between 100 and 200 bases long. The advantage of this method is that specialized microarrays can easily be fabricated to search for specific genes. However, given the size of the spots, there are limits on the number of probes that can be put onto one spot of the microarray. For this reason, the use of smaller probes is generally preferred, and these are put on the chip using photolithographic techniques adapted from semiconductor technology. The probes are built 'bottom-up' and in parallel in the same way that circuits are, so that nucleotides are added to multiple growing chains simultaneously. A 'spot' ('well' or 'cell') on a gene chip can contain a thousand probes for one specific gene.

After the mRNA samples (control and experiment) are reverse transcribed into cDNA, labelled (dyed) and allowed to hybridize with the probes on the microarray or gene chip in the form of cRNA, lasers are used to produce an emission signal for each dye. It is not yet possible for computers to be linked directly to gene chips and microarrays so that the amount of mRNA in a sample can be read directly from the probe cells. DNA probes and mRNA fragments are far too small to be read in this manner. Instead, the array or gene chip has to be converted into a fluorescent image which is sufficiently detailed at the pixel level to allow inferences to be made about the quantity of sample in a cell. Confocal array scanners are currently the most popular method of measuring the fluorescence. A gene chip probe cell is currently beween 25 μm and 50 μm, and pixel sizes used by confocal lasers are about 5 μm. Confocal lasers can therefore produce six-by-six or eight-by-eight pixel images of a gene chip well or spot. Each pixel will have a certain colour attached to it, and the overall 'colour' of the spot or cell is determined by the colour of the individual pixels making up the spot. For instance, if two colours are used (say, red for experimental mRNA sample and green for control mRNA sample), and cRNA of both samples hybridize with the probes of a cell, all pixels will give off a yellow/orange diffraction pattern. If, however, mRNA of only one sample is present and hybridizes with the probes in a cell, a diffraction pattern which represents red or green will be produced which is broken down by the pixel matrix (Figure 2.6 (1)). The outermost pixels are removed from analysis and the intensity of pixels plotted to arrive at an average intensity value for the cell as a whole to determine whether enough sample is present in a cell.

Quantitiation (converting fluorescence intensities into amounts of sample) usually results in large numbers that are conventionally converted into $\log_2$ ratios. For instance, if after laser analysis there are 200 transcripts of red cRNA for a gene and 10 000 transcripts of green cRNA, $\log_2(10\,000/200) = 5.64$. If the expression values are identical, the result is 0. Minus $\log_2$ values would signify more red cRNA than green. Such $\log_2$ ratios are easier to work with as well as provide absolute values, even if they have to be subsequently normalized to overcome skewed frequency distributions. Interpreting $\log_2$ ratios can, however, be difficult. Also, determining how reliable both $\log_2$ ratios and raw intensity values are is difficult. Different amounts of the two samples and of labelling concentrations may have been used, for instance, which will affect the quantitiation process.

Alternatively, Affymetrix gene chips use a *perfect-match/mismatch* strategy to help identify the reliability of the readings as well as produce an *absolute call* value for each gene which expresses whether the gene probed for is 'present', 'absent' or 'marginal' (Figure 2.6 (2)). Affymetrix use two types of probe in a cell: a 25-nucleotide sequence which is identical to a fragment of a sample mRNA and a 25-nucleotide sequence which is identical to the probe except that the middle base is different. If the

(1)

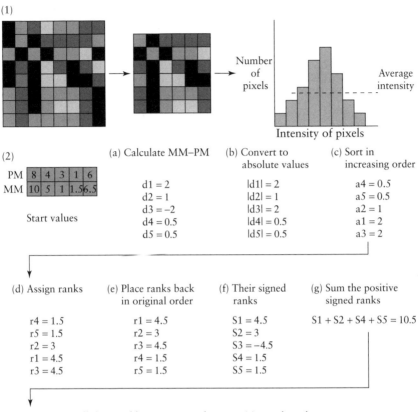

(2)

PM | 8 | 4 | 3 | 1 | 6
MM | 10 | 5 | 1 | 1.5 | 6.5

Start values

(a) Calculate MM–PM

d1 = 2
d2 = 1
d3 = −2
d4 = 0.5
d5 = 0.5

(b) Convert to absolute values

|d1| = 2
|d2| = 1
|d3| = 2
|d4| = 0.5
|d5| = 0.5

(c) Sort in increasing order

a4 = 0.5
a5 = 0.5
a2 = 1
a1 = 2
a3 = 2

(d) Assign ranks

r4 = 1.5
r5 = 1.5
r2 = 3
r1 = 4.5
r3 = 4.5

(e) Place ranks back in original order

r1 = 4.5
r2 = 3
r3 = 4.5
r4 = 1.5
r5 = 1.5

(f) Their signed ranks

S1 = 4.5
S2 = 3
S3 = −4.5
S4 = 1.5
S5 = 1.5

(g) Sum the positive signed ranks

S1 + S2 + S4 + S5 = 10.5

(h) Enumerate all the possible outcomes and sum positive ranks only:

						Sum
1	−1.5	−1.5	−3	−4.5	−4.5	0
2	1.5	−1.5	−3	−4.5	−4.5	1.5
3	−1.5	1.5	−3	−4.5	−4.5	1.5
4	−1.5	−1.5	3	−4.5	−4.5	3
			...			
26	−1.5	−1.5	3	4.5	4.5	12
27	1.5	1.5	3	4.5	−4.5	10.5
28	1.5	1.5	3	−4.5	4.5	10.5
29	1.5	1.5	−3	4.5	4.5	12
30	1.5	−1.5	3	4.5	4.5	13.5
31	−1.5	1.5	3	4.5	4.5	13.5
32	1.5	1.5	3	4.5	4.5	15

(i) All signed ranks above 10.5 are given the weight 1 (5 in the table) and signed ranks equal to 10.5 (4) are given the weight 0.5. Now calculate the p value:

$$P(10.5) = (1*5 + 0.5*4)/32$$
$$= 0.21875$$

(j) Since the p value is not significant (not below 0.05), this gene is absent.

Figure 2.6   Affymetrix gene chip technology

base in the middle of a probe sequence is not complementary to the base in the middle of the sample sequence, the repulsion forces between just these two bases should be sufficient to ensure that the sample sequence does not hybridize with the probe sequence. Mismatch probes therefore allow for checks on non-specific cross-hybridization in the sample. That is, outside of the human body mRNA nucleotides are not always guaranteed to bind to their complementary base pairs, due to heat differences and degradation, for instance. These mismatch probes are also used to generate absolute call values in that the fewer mismatches there are, the more confidence one has in the accuracy of the perfect matched figures. In Figure 2.6 (2) a gene is probed across several 'probe pairs' (typically 10–15 on Affymetrix gene chips), where each pair is made up of 'perfect-match' probe sequences and 'mismatch' probe sequences. To determine whether a gene is present in a sample, Wilcoxon's Signed Rank Test is used. Imagine there are five probe pairs for a gene (each probe pair consists of a perfect match and a mismatch beneath it) and the values are as indicated in Figure 2.6 (2), where these values represent the number of samples hybridized in each of the cells. The first step is to calculate the difference between each pair (a), followed by a conversion to absolute values (b), which are then sorted and ranked (c, d). The ranked values are placed back in their original order (e) and re-allocated their signs (f). The sum of the positive signed ranks is calculated (g) and a full enumeration of all possible signed outcomes is listed (h), with only positive ranks summed. All signed ranks above the sum calculated at step (g) are given the weight 1 and equal to the sum the weight 0.5 (i). The p value is then calculated as the sum of the weighted values divided by the total number of enumerated outcomes. If the value is below 0.045 a value of 'present' is attached to the gene, if the value is above 0.055 a value of 'absent' is returned, and otherwise 'marginal'.

Gene chips now exist for measuring the expression levels of all genes in the human genome. They can also be used to check whether genes are being expressed in specific tissue and which genes are expressed in response to drugs. One particular application of gene chips and microarrays is in the identification of single nucleotide polymorphisms (SNPs) that express common genetic variances among people, caused by a single nucleotide change every 300 bases or so in both the coding and non-coding parts of the human genome. For a nucleotide change to be an SNP, it should occur in at least 1 per cent of the population, and it is believed that, while SNPs do not affect the normal function of cells, they do affect the way that individuals react to drugs or predispose individuals to certain diseases. Microarrays and gene chips can be purpose-designed to identify SNPs and detect their presence in individuals.

While DNA arrays and gene chips are among the most exciting genomic tools to have been developed within the last few years, it has to be remembered that mRNA levels do not always correlate with protein levels. It is not currently known how much mRNA actually makes it to protein.

Alternative splice variants of genes that are not measured on a DNA chip mean that a gene may not be accurately measured. Also, DNA chips cannot identify post-translational modifications of a protein. However, perhaps the biggest problem with DNA chips concerns current gene expression analysis techniques. The sheer volume of data (gene expression datasets can be several megabytes) leads to the need for fast analytical tools; but more importantly, there are many more attributes (genes) than records (samples). Typically, 12 000 to 25 000 genes are measured for each sample (subject or individual), and only 50 to 100 samples are collected. In database terms this leads to a hugely sparse data space. Gene expression analysis (G) can be defined to be concerned with selecting a small subset of relevant genes from the original set of genes (the S problem) as well as combining individual genes in either the original or smaller subsets of genes to identify important causal and classificatory relationships (the C problem). That is, $G = S + C$. In later chapters it will be shown how artificial intelligence techniques are making promising progress in analysing gene expression data and mining the data for useful knowledge.

The analysis problem becomes even more acute when dealing with temporal gene expression data, i.e. the repeated application of DNA chips to measure the transcriptomic state of an individual over time. So far it has been assumed that DNA chips are used to measure an individual just once and that the database will consist of several samples, measured once, where each sample falls in a clearly designated and independently observed class (e.g. a cancerous sample versus a normal one). Imagine that an individual cancer patient's mRNA is measured at time 0 and then a drug added which, it is believed, will 'cure' the patient. The individual's mRNA is measured after 30 min, then 1 h, then 2 h, then 4 h, etc., to see how the drug is affecting gene expression of the immune system and whether cancerous cells are being targeted for attack by the immune system. What is of interest here is the network of gene activation over time, as expressed not just for one patient but for several patients. The task is to 'reverse engineer' this gene network from not just one dataset but several. Reverse engineering means identifying which genes at one time point affect which other genes at the next time point. Given the large numbers of genes measured, if each gene is allowed to affect every other gene, a search space will rapidly be generated that is too complex for computers to analyse. If a gene at one time-step is restricted to affecting only five other genes at the next time step, or a gene at a subsequent time-step to be affected by only five other genes at the previous time-step, the question is how to identify just these small numbers of affected or affecting genes from the huge number measured. Reverse engineering gene networks from gene expression data, where there is confidence that the correct causally influencing and causally influenced genes have been identified, is one of the biggest unsolved problems in bioinformatics.

Ethical considerations

There is also an ethical dimension to gene expression analysis. First, measuring the gene expression of an individual gives us information on not just that individual but also that individual's closest relatives. So while an individual may well permit their gene expression to be measured and a genetic profile for that individual to be stored in a database, there are fundamental questions about the rights of that individual's relatives to have information about their genetic profiles not stored in a database. Identifying through gene expression analysis that an individual has a predisposition to a particular inheritable disease provides information about other members of that individual's family. Secondly, while it may be acceptable to measure the gene expression of individuals who are suffering from a disease, there are fundamental questions concerning the scope of gene expression analysis. Should embryonic stem cells be monitored for gene expression, for instance, so that important information is obtained about how cells are differentiated during the early stages of fetal development? One of the most puzzling of all mysteries in biology is the way in which, from one fertilized cell, a multi-trillion cellular organism called a human results, where billions of cells have somehow 'agreed' to express only certain genes that allow them to form tissue and cooperate with each other. The fertilized cell and its daughter cells after initial division within a few hours are *totipotent*, i.e. they have the ability to become any cell in the body. After about four days some of these cells become a blastocyst (hollow sphere) and have lost their totipotency, whereas the other cells inside the blastocyst form an inner cell mass. These inner cells are *pluripotent* in that they have the ability to become one of several different types of cell. After further division pluripotent cells become *multipotent*, whereby a multipotent brain cell, for instance, has the ability to become any one of the different types of brain cell (Figure 2.7).

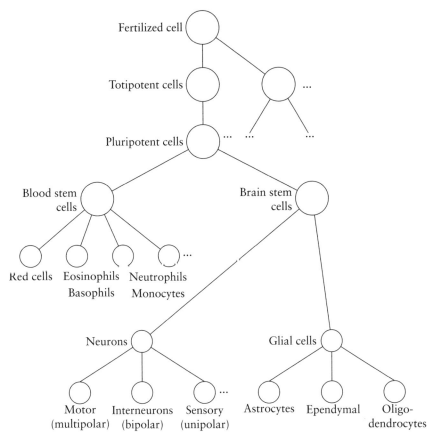

Figure 2.7   Embryonic stem cells

Currently there are two methods for developing pluripotent cells: from inner cell mass at the blastocyst stage and from fetal tissue from terminated pregnancies. While DNA chips provide an unprecedented opportunity to measure early gene expression (within a few hours of conception), this may mean that embryos are 'farmed' for research purposes. The promise of stem cells lies in their possible ability, when located next to damaged tissue, to become one of the cells in that tissue by expressing the same genes as those expressed in the tissue. The mechanisms whereby this happens are not known, but the potential to repair parts of the body where cells no longer divide in sufficient numbers to overcome damage (such as the brain or liver) is huge. However, before stem cells can be used there needs to be an understanding of their gene expression and differentiation mechanisms. Different countries are taking different ethical and legislative stances on this important ethical topic.

2.4 Proteome

Secondary and tertiary structure prediction

Proteins are the end result of translation of mRNA by ribosomes. Once protein sequences of amino acids leave the ribosomes they fold in complex ways to achieve a 'native' state or conformation in the cell. The native state of a protein is a highly stable three-dimensional structure that helps determine its biological function. In other words, a protein cannot function unless it folds in the right way. For instance, catalytic proteins must fold in such a way that they can lock onto another molecule (substrate), thereby lowering the energy threshold required to start a reaction in the substrate. Once the reaction takes place, the catalytic protein is released to find other molecules to attach to so that further reactions can take place. If the catalytic protein misfolds, it will not be able to start the catalytic reaction. In particular, the *active site* of the protein which locks onto the appropriate section of the target molecule (the *substrate*) to start a reaction may not be revealed and so the protein cannot function.

Protein misfolding is associated with several diseases, and to understand the nature of the disease at the molecular level involves understanding the way that amino acids both locally and distantly affect the folding. That is, while it may not be possible to predict how a specific sequence of amino acids folds locally, once it folds it comes into contact with other regions of amino acids elsewhere in the sequence. Folding is determined by the chemical and physical properties of the amino acids making up the protein, but such chemical and physical explanations of folding have to take into account 'long distance' relationships between different parts of the same sequence. Determining the way that proteins fold into specific shapes is called the 'protein folding problem'. Laboratory experiments have shown that if a protein is gently denatured (that is, unfolded by, say, raising the temperature or changing the salt concentration of the surrounding fluid) and then allowed to refold, it resumes its original structure, thereby demonstrating that the ability of the protein to fold into its correct shape is intrinsic (all the information required to fold a protein is in the protein constituents).

While one obvious use of computers in bioinformatics is the storing of DNA sequence information and constructing the correct DNA sequences from fragments identified by restriction enzymes (enzymes which break up the DNA at certain points), protein sequences and the polypeptide[3]

---

[3] The term 'peptide' is used to refer to short sequences of amino acids, while the term 'polypeptide' refers to sequences of length 50 or more.

sequences that make up that protein also need to be stored. New protein sequences are being added to protein databases as a result of analysing mRNA sequences, where redundantly transcribed DNA (introns) have been removed, and by translating codons via the genetic code into letters of the amino acid alphabet. However, these linear sequences of amino acids (polypeptide sequence) do not tell us anything about the *structure* of the protein or how it folds. The protein folding problem is important because it takes a lot of effort to determine the structure of an actual protein. A real protein has to be to denatured (unfolded) so that its amino acid sequence can be described, but denaturing a protein *and* sequencing its amino acid content are much more difficult than simply denaturing a protein. In the act of denaturing the structure of the protein is affected so that information is lost about the structure as amino acids making up the protein are sequenced. Identifying the structure of a protein requires complex measurement, typically through X-ray crystallography or nuclear magnetic resonance (NMR) spectroscopy techniques, neither of which may be readily available to biologists. In any case, not all proteins are susceptible to crystallization, and NMR is constrained to deal with small proteins because of the computational costs involved in trying to model complex proteins. Finally, to determine the structure of a protein means removing it from its natural environment – the cell or organism. There is no guarantee that a protein being experimentally investigated *in vitro* will have the same structure as *in vivo*. As a consequence, the number of experimentally determined protein sequences is far fewer than the number of protein sequences that have been 'translated' by a computer from DNA and mRNA sequences.

The structure of a real protein is conventionally described in four ways (Figure 2.8). The *primary* structure of a protein (Figure 2.8(a)) is the sequence of amino acids produced at ribosomes. Since there are 20 amino acids, the primary structure describes the precise order of amino acids in the protein. The *secondary* structure of a protein (Figure 2.8(b)) describes those parts of the primary structure (subsequences of amino acids) that fold into regular and repeated patterns, such as α-*helices*, β-*sheets*, or *turns* (see Figure 2.9 for conventional computer-generated graphical ways of describing secondary structure). The *tertiary* structure (Figure 2.8(c)) consists of those elements of the secondary structure that build more complex units, such as an $\alpha-\beta$ *motif*, and provide a three-dimensional shape of the protein. The tertiary structure of enzymes is typically a compact, globular shape, for instance. Finally, many proteins consist of more than one polypeptide chain. The *quaternary* structure of a protein (Figure 2.8(d)) is a description of how several separate polypeptide sequences have come together to form a complex protein.

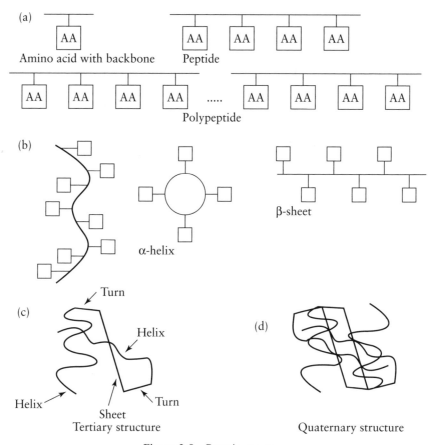

Figure 2.8   Protein structure

For instance, human haemoglobin consists of four separate polypeptides that come together to form a complex molecule that takes up oxygen from the lungs and delivers it to the cells of the body. These four peptides result from the translation of four separate genes. For experimental biologists, identifying all four levels of structure from an actual protein is very difficult, since not all parts of the protein are available for analysis. A real protein has to be dissected into smaller parts so that amino acids hidden by folds are revealed. There is therefore a great need to work from primary structures of proteins (as revealed by mRNA) to the three-dimensional and quaternary structure of the protein. Currently, this task is proving a great challenge to computer scientists because of the complexity of predicting secondary, tertiary and quaternary structures from primary structures. Folding arises because of basic charges (attraction and repulsion) of atoms and molecules, and modelling these for long sequences of amino acids is proving difficult.

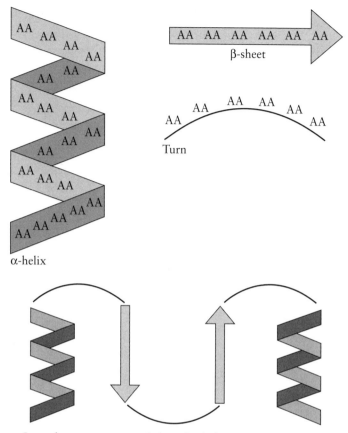

α-helix

β-sheet

Turn

Secondary structure consisting of α-helix, turn, β-sheet, turn, β-sheet, turn, α-helix

Figure 2.9   Computer visualization of a secondary structure

There are currently three approaches to protein folding prediction. *Comparative modelling* (also known as modelling by homology or knowledge-based modelling) uses structural data from experimentally determined protein sequences. An amino acid alignment is first made between protein sequences with unknown structure (typically derived from DNA or mRNA translation by the computer) with protein sequences with known structure. Then where the alignment agrees, the conformation of the sequence with known structure is allocated to the sequence with unknown structure for that part of the alignment. The main problem with comparative modelling is that there can be significant similarities between two proteins with known structure where the structures are significantly different from each other. Similarity of primary sequence is therefore no guarantee of similarity of structure and therefore of function. Similarly, there are also examples of two proteins with known structure with similar function where the primary sequence information is significantly different in each sequence. Typically a threshold value of 30 per cent sequence identity is required to be exceeded before two sequences are considered homologous for modelling. While this figure may appear to be low, the argument is that the three-dimensional structure of proteins is conserved to a greater extent than the primary sequence. That is, a high degree of primary sequence similarity between a protein with known structure and a protein with unknown structure is not needed, since the function of a protein, as given by its structure, is more likely to be preserved through its shape than its amino acid sequence. The homologies being searched for are assumed to reflect structurally conserved regions of the protein.

Fold recognition, or *threading*, techniques are similar to homology modelling techniques but use a database of proteins with known structure and folds (called templates) against which to compare the protein of unknown structure. A scoring function is used to rank the folds and the folds with the best scores are then adopted for the protein with unknown folds and structure.

The final method is *ab initio*, where a structure is predicted for a protein with unknown structure by using physical principles of folding. One of the main assumptions of this method is that the native structure of a protein reflects its global free energy minimum, and the task of *ab initio* methods is to search the space of possible conformations of the amino acids (residues) making up a sequence to find optimal conformations that achieve low energy levels. While some *ab initio* methods work at the atomic level for residues, in practice residues are modelled using only a few interaction centres within the residue. Many molecular dynamics optimization methods now exist, using lattice-based enumerations and diffusion equation methods. The basic approach is to minimize the energy of the system, add a structural change, minimize the energy, add a structural change, and so on. *Ab initio* methods may have to be used when suitable template structures are not available.

Problems with *ab initio* methods include a minor conformational change at one residue having major implications for the entire sequence, which may not be captured by the simulation models used. For instance, a bond between two residues may be rotated for local minimization of energy, but given that the structure as a whole is three-dimensional there may be unfavourable effects on the whole structure that cannot be captured by the simulation. Also, the complexity involved in predicting the structure of a large protein may be too hard for a computer. Nor has it escaped the attention of some researchers that large proteins naturally fold within seconds of translation, whereas computer models take hours or even days to predict the structure of less complex proteins.

Protein folding is perhaps the biggest problem in bioinformatics currently. Even if good techniques and methods for predicting the structure of proteins from primary sequences are discovered, this may not reveal anything about how the biological function or activity of that protein is carried out. There is also increasing interest in the actual stage-by-stage process by which a protein naturally folds to identify causes of misfolding. Current protein folding methods may not actually reflect this natural folding process. Yet there is increasing evidence that many diseases, such as Alzheimer's, cystic fibrosis, sickle cell anaemia, bovine spongiform encephalopathy (BSE) and its human equivalent Creutzfeldt–Jakob disease (CJD), are due to misfolding. It is currently estimated that of the several hundred thousand protein sequences stored in databanks (derived from DNA and mRNA), only about 1 per cent have an experimentally determined structure. As genome projects provide increasingly more protein sequences in their databases, this mismatch between proteins of known structure and unknown structure is bound to grow. *In silico* methods of accurately predicting the structure of proteins are still at an early stage of development and present one of the most profound challenges in bioinformatics.

Protein identification

Another current challenge in bioinformatics is to determine how large the human proteome (the total collection of all proteins produced by the genome) actually is. While many prokaryotic cells have small numbers of genes in comparison to the human cells (about 5000, typically), there is little evidence of significant alternative splicing. However, post-translational modification of proteins as they emerge from the ribosomes may increase the number of proteins so that anywhere between 10 000 and 20 000 proteins are actually produced by a prokaryotic cell. For a human (eukaryotic) cell containing 30 000 genes, it is currently estimated that each gene can be alternatively spliced anywhere between three and 100 times. Even assuming the lower figure, that gives about 90 000 different polypeptide sequences. However, several different types of post-translational modification can be carried out, such as cleavage of polypeptide sequences at different points to give different proteins, including removal of the initial methionine residue. Many proteins are *inactive precursors* that are activated under appropriate physiological conditions. Their task is to be present in the body should a situation arise when they are suddenly required, for instance, enzymes for forming clots in the blood in the case of a wound. Such *proproteins* are typically activated by the removal of certain amino acids at the ends of a protein, allowing the protein to function by revealing the active site of the protein. The task of proteomics is to identify not just all the different proteins that can be produced by a genome but also to detect those proteins that are associated with disease because of misfolding of proteins or different amounts of protein.

The biggest problem for proteomics currently is a suitable technology for measuring the variety and abundance of protein in a cell or organism. The most common form of measurement is *protein electrophoresis*. Proteins have an electrical charge, and the basic method is to place all protein from a sample on a gel and apply an electrical current to the gel so that the proteins move to different parts of the gel depending on their electrical charge; they then form bands that indicate the relative proportion of each protein fraction. Proteins are separated because at some point in the migration there is no net charge, and the protein is then stationary. While this form of measurement is appropriate when comparing different samples, the technology does not allow for the individual identification of proteins in a sample. Also, small proteins move through the gel more quickly than large proteins and may end up in regions of the gel that cannot be measured accurately because of smearing or distortion. Many proteins also react unpredictably with the gel and may migrate to wrong parts of the gel matrix. Gel electrophoresis also requires a great deal of expert human manipulation, leading to increased possibility of error. However, automated protein identification techniques using gels are increasingly appearing on the market. Nevertheless, gel-based techniques by themselves may not be sufficiently accurate to identify individual proteins.

New techniques being explored currently for individual protein identification include peptide-mass fingerprinting and peptide sequencing. The former uses *proteases* (special proteins that cut other proteins) to dissect specific proteins into fragments that have a unique 'fingerprint' when subjected to NMR spectroscopy techniques. The correct identification of these fingerprints requires access to a database of protein fragments and their signatures under specific NMR spectroscopy conditions. However, as more proteins and their fragments are included in such databases, the chances of finding unique fingerprints begin to worsen! Ideally, it would be helpful if a protein could be sequenced in the same way that a gene can be sequenced (through complementary base pairing techniques). Amino acids do not have complements, however. Peptide sequencing attempts to identify the amino acids of a protein or protein fragment either by working from one end of the fragment (*terminus* sequencing), one residue at a time, by cutting the residue from the sequence and then using complex methods for identifying the residue that has been cut off, or if the terminus is not visible by cutting the sequence into a number of fragments and then identifying each residue, as before (*internal* sequencing). Again, NMR or other mass spectrometry techniques are used for identifying residues, and many biologists do not have easy access to such facilities. Also, fragmentation processes are not sufficiently advanced to ensure that a protein is cut at the correct locations.

High-throughput peptide sequencing analogous to nucleotide high-throughput sequencing is a fundamental requirement for identifying novel proteins and novel ways in which proteins are translated from their mRNA sequences. The future bioinformatics problem, once high-throughput protein identification techniques are made available, is to map the actual proteins and their sequences found in cells with genome databases. Given the variety of alternate splicing of mRNA and post-translational modifications, the identification of exactly which gene is the source for which protein sequences is not likely to be an easy task, especially given the redundancy in the genetic code (several different ways of DNA mapping onto amino acid).

2.5 Interference technology, viruses and the immune system

Interference technology

Proteomics is considered one of the most important ways of understanding gene function. That is, even if a gene is fully sequenced and located on a chromosome, this does not mean that there is a full understanding of the gene unless it is known what its translated products do. So even if there is full knowledge of a genome and full knowledge of all the proteins derivable from that genome, a full understanding of the genome and proteome will only come with a detailed understanding of how genes affect other genes through proteins, of how proteins affect other proteins. While the genome is static, in that once it is characterized it can be assumed to be constant, the proteome is dynamic and reflects the state of the cell and the conditions under which it survives. Some proteins are produced only when the cell's environment is stressed (e.g. by heating). It is possible that there is a specific stress gene for that condition that only comes on when the stress condition is apparent, but it is also possible that the cell deals with the stress either by producing more quantity of a protein or by modifying a product of an already expressed gene. One way to study the effects of proteins is through 'knock-out' technology that effectively silences genes. If genes can be silenced under controlled conditions, the effects of the absence of the gene on the proteome can be studied. While one method for silencing genes is to look upstream of a gene and at its transcription regulatory elements to see if promoter and enhancer regions can be blocked, not enough is known currently about these regions to determine effective gene silencing mechanisms at the transcriptional level. However, *interference* technology provides a mechanism for regulating the translation of mRNA even if transcription takes place.

Antisense technology is an mRNA interference technology that blocks the translation of 'sense' mRNA (see Figure 1.5) and is based on the idea of introducing an antisense gene or antisense RNA into cells. The effect of antisense technology has been known for over 20 years but its mechanisms were not understood. Introducing a short piece of antisense RNA, that is, a sequence that is complementary to part of an mRNA sequence, produced the obvious result that the gene giving rise to the mRNA was silenced due to its mRNA being partly double-stranded when the antisense RNA paired with the appropriate sequences of complementary bases in the transcribed mRNA. Such double-stranding was assumed to prevent the ribosomes from effectively translating the sequence of amino acids in the mRNA. In other words, it was assumed that the ribosomes 'jammed' when the mRNA transcript was found to contain double-stranded codons rather than the linear sequence of single-stranded codons expected. However, it was also found that introducing a *sense* RNA subsequence (that is, a subsequence that is identical to part of the mRNA) produced the same silencing effect. Sense RNA cannot pair with sense mRNA, since the bases are identical. Finally, it was also discovered that introducing a small section of *double-stranded RNA* was more effective at silencing the target gene than introducing either a sense or antisense RNA strand. To understand the mechanisms at work, viruses and the immune system will need to be explored.

Viruses and the immune system

A virus is not a living entity or cell, since it lacks many of the essential components of a cell, such as translation machinery and cellular transport systems. It is between 20 and 100 times smaller than a typical single cell organism and attacks all types of cell or organism. Viruses that attack bacteria are called *bacteriophages*. A virus is a piece of genetic sequence (either DNA or RNA) with some proteins, wrapped up in a protein coat (*capsid*) and with the ability to recognize specific prokaryotic and eukaryotic cells through sites on the capsid that are complementary to receptors on the target cell. When a virus recognizes the cell it is specifically tuned for, it attaches itself to the cell and injects its genetic material (DNA or RNA sequence together with any viral proteins). The cell processes (transcribes and translates) the viral genetic material which contains the information on how to make components of the virus (such as the capsid, recognition sites and the genetic material). As the components are produced, they assemble into complete copies of the original virus (*virions*) and are released from the cell to target other cells. The host cell's transcription and translation machinery may be so overcome with the task of reproducing the virus that it stops making the essential components required to enable it to survive, or the virions are released from the cell by puncturing a hole in the membrane of the cell, thereby killing the cell as its contents leak out.

Viruses come in many different forms, and the *Baltimore Classification* identifies viruses according to the nature of the genetic material they contain. Viruses can contain, for example, (a) double-stranded DNA (typically 5000 base pairs (bp) to 300 000 bp), (b) single-stranded DNA, (c) double-stranded RNA, (d) positive sense single-stranded RNA, and (e) negative sense single-stranded RNA. Of these, the positive sense single-stranded RNA class is the best known to humans, causing the common cold (*rhinoviruses*) and meningitis (*enterovirus*). A viral infection is dangerous to an organism because, if the infection goes unchecked, a sufficiently large number of cells can be killed which leads to the organism as a whole dying. An example of HIV (human immunodeficiency virus, considered to be the main cause of AIDS (Acquired Immunodeficiency Syndrome)), is provided in Figure 2.10.

The HIV virion consists of two single-stranded negative sense RNA sequences (about 9000 bases each) containing at least nine genes, plus three proteins – a reverse transcriptase, an integrase and a protease (Figure 2.10(a)). The HIV virion attaches itself to lymphocytes (helper and killer T cells) of the immune system through the CD4 and CCR5 receptors

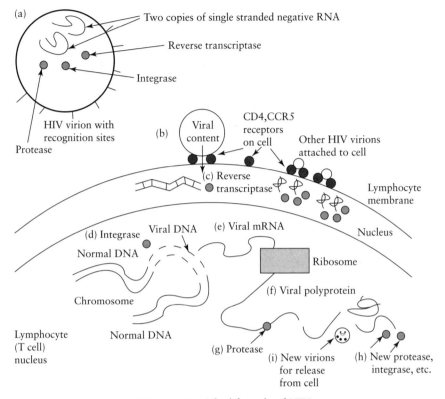

Figure 2.10   The life cycle of HIV

on the surface of the cell (Figure 2.10(b)). The viral content (RNA and proteins) is injected into the cell, and the reverse transcriptase makes a positive copy of one of the negative strand viral RNA to form a double strand (Figure 2.10(c)). The viral integrase takes the double strand into the nucleus and splices it into the cell's DNA (Figure 2.10(d)). Normal cellular machinery then transcribes (Figure 2.10(e)) and translates the viral mRNA to form one long viral polyprotein sequence (Figure 2.10(f)). The third viral protein, protease (Figure 2.10(g)) has the task of cleaving the viral polyprotein into constituent parts (new copies of viral protein, capsid, etc., Figure 2.10(h)) so that new virions can be assembled for further infection (Figure 2.10(i)).

The human immune system has developed a number of methods for detecting and eradicating viruses and other *pathogens* (any disease-producing agent including bacteria) by activating both an *innate* and *adaptive* response. Innate responses are general responses to a limited number of pathogens and include *phagocytes* (scavenger cells) and *macrophages* (either fixed to specific locations in the body or circulating with the blood) that 'swallow' whole pathogens or clear up debris. Such cells are directed to pathogens through the stimulation of *antibodies* (immunoglobulins) in response to *antigens* and other substances produced by the pathogen. Also part of the innate response are the *natural killer* cells that destroy cells in the body that have been infected to prevent the infection from spreading. If the innate system cannot deal with the pathogen, the adaptive system takes over. One important part of the adaptive system consists of *lymphocytes* (white blood cells) binding approximately to pathogens. This can result in *B-lymphocytes* (cells produced in bone marrow) producing antibodies to bring the pathogen to the attention of macrophages and phagocytes for destruction, or cloning themselves in large numbers with even more specialized binding mechanisms so that they can inactivate the pathogens directly. Approximate binding and cloning by B-cells provides us with the ability to identify and deal with any new pathogen. However, since approximate binding and cloning can lead to the production of B-lymphocytes that inadvertently attach themselves to healthy *self-cells* (cells that are part of the body and not foreign to the body), the immune system requires *helper T-cells* (cells produced in the thymus) to co-stimulate B-cells only if the B-cell is not attached to a healthy (non-antigen presenting) self-cell. This is particularly important in the case of viruses that have infected self-cells. Such infected cells produce fragments of the virus on their surface through the use of *major histocompatability* (*MHC*) *molecules*. If helper T-cells recognize these viral fragments on the surface of self-cells, it produces a co-stimulus to the B-cell which then destroys the infected cell. One of the critical properties of HIV is that it attacks these helper T-cells (Figure 2.10). If these immune system cells become infected, they can no longer provide the co-stimulation required for B-cells to work. The immune system then becomes sufficiently weakened (Acquired Immunodeficiency Syndrome – AIDS) that any pathogen that would normally be non-dangerous to us becomes lethal. With this basic understanding of viral and immune system behaviour, gene silencing can be described in more detail.

Post-transcriptional gene silencing in multicellular organisms is considered to be an evolutionary conserved, single cell defence mechanism for dealing with foreign genes and RNA introduced typically by a virus. That is, before multicellular organisms – with their complex immune systems requiring the cooperation of many different types of cell – developed from single-cell organisms, such single-cell organisms had to fight pathogens on their own and without the help of other cells. Both positive-sense and negative-sense RNA are produced by different types of virus, and the cell had to find a mechanism to prevent their expression. Also, double-stranded RNA can be produced by viruses using reverse transcriptase. Since all three types of sequence were found to silence genes in multicellular organisms, the current hypothesis is that the underlying gene silencing mechanisms reflect the manner in which single cells prevented infection.

The current model of interference is that an enzyme called *Dicer* (Figure 2.11(a)) takes the introduced double-stranded RNA and cuts it into small (20–25 bp) sequences called *small interfering RNA* (siRNA) (Figure 2.11 (b)), which in turn – after separating into single strands – bind to an RNA-inducing silencing complex (*RISC*) (Figure 2.11(c)).These

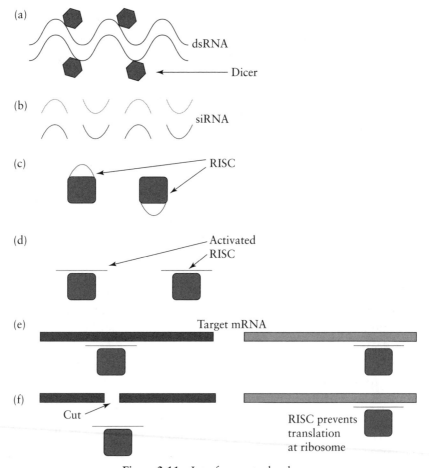

Figure 2.11   Interference technology

become activated when the siRNA unfolds (Figure 2.11(d)) and the activated RISCs then target mRNA transcripts through complementary base pairing (Figure 2.11(e)). If transcripts containing the appropriate complementary sequences are found, they are cut or the RISC binds to the transcript to prevent translation of the transcript at the ribosome (Figure 2.11(f)). In some organisms a 'spreading' effect has been found, whereby the cut mRNA is copied to form secondary siRNA for use in RISCs. This copy process is used to explain why introducing a sense RNA strand can also lead to gene silencing. However, for effective gene silencing, dsRNA is rarely used, since such strands can trigger an anti-viral response from the immune system leading to the cell's death. Instead, siRNA is currently used to silence genes. Such siRNA can be produced synthetically and injected into cells, or they can be transported into the cell with the help of viral 'vectors' (safe viruses that have been genetically engineered to contain a DNA sequence which, when inserted into a cell and transcribed, produce the siRNA). Current research points to whole genome functional analysis being possible in the near future, where all genes are individually screened by siRNA and the resulting transcriptomes and proteomes measured to identify the effects. It is currently unclear as to exactly what sort of bioinformatics resource will be needed to support systematic functional analysis of genomes. Also, current research into RNA interference (RNAi) technology is directed towards fighting viral diseases (the production of siRNA that prevents viral mRNA from being translated) and silencing cancer-associated genes (e.g. siRNA to silence cell division). Many of these problems are so complex that standard modelling and simulation tools may not be adequate. Novel methods and techniques may have to be developed to take bioinformatics into the next generation.

2.6 Summary of chapter

1 The major problems in bioinformatics can be distinguished according to the areas into which these problems fall: genomics, transcriptomics and proteomics.

2 Current problems in the post-genomic era deal with sequence analysis and phylogenetic analysis to make clear the relationships between organisms as the number of fully sequences genomes grows. However, there are problems in being able to compare organisms in such a way that clear and unambiguous phylogenetic relationships emerge.

3   Transcriptomics is a relatively new problem area arising from recent technological advances in DNA arrays (microarrays and gene chips). The major problems here, apart from obtaining the data, is the analysis of the data given the large number of genes measured for a comparatively small number of samples. Novel techniques may need to be developed to reverse engineer gene networks from temporal data so that the interrelationships between genes are clearly identified.

4   Protein folding prediction is one of the oldest known problems in proteomics and hence bioinformatics. Problems exist in sequencing a protein without affecting its nature, and techniques for predicting the structure of proteins from their linear sequence need improving.

5   A new problem area concerns interference technology and the way that genes can be silenced to measure their effect. Of great interest is the application of interference technology to immune systems, since it is by observing the effect of switching off genes and interfering with genes of the immune system that a greater understanding will be obtained of how the body fights infections, thereby leading to future drugs that can be more carefully targeted for particular viruses.

6   Finally, embryonic stem cell research provides a novel way to understand cell differentiation for possible future cures of diseases currently believed to be untreatable. There are, however, ethical considerations with regard to embryonic stem cell research that will need discussion before approval can be given to such research.

2.7 Further reading

Baldi, P. and Hatfield, G.W. (2002) *DNA Microarrays and Gene Expression*, Cambridge University Press.

Coico, R., Sunshine, G. and Benjamini, E. (2003) *Immunology: A Short Course*, 5th edn, Wiley–Liss.

Mount, D.W. (2001) *Bioinformatics: Sequence and Genome Analysis*, Cold Spring Harbor Laboratory Press.

Parson, A.B. (2004) *The Proteus Effect: Stem Cells and Their Promise*, National Academies Press.

Ridley, M. (2003) *Evolution*, 3rd edn, Blackwell.

Sternberg, M.J.E. (ed) (1996) *Protein Structure Prediction*, IRL Press.

3

Introduction to Artificial Intelligence and Computer Science

3.1 Introduction to search

One of the most fundamental tasks in computer science is *search*. Many problems can be converted into search problems, including the simple problem of adding two numbers, such as 2 + 2. The search representation of this problem is whether there exists a number (in this case, 4) that can be reached from the original statement of the problem. To determine an alignment between two DNA sequences can also be regarded as a search problem: given the starting point of two sequences, find a solution that minimizes as much as possible the differences between the two sequences. The development of search techniques received a major boost with the formalization of graph theory, with graphs being defined formally and precisely in terms of nodes and arcs that connect them. A labelled graph has one or more descriptors called labels on each node that distinguish that node from all other nodes in the graph. In a *state space search* these labels identify *states* during a problem-solving process. Also, the arcs (connections between nodes) can be labelled to represent some relationship between nodes. Usually these labels represent weights, or costs involved in moving between one state and another. A graph is *directed* if the arcs have arrows, signifying directionality.

In a state space representation of a computational problem, the nodes of the graph represent partial solutions to the problem and the arcs

Intelligent Bioinformatics   Edward Keedwell and Ajit Narayanan
© 2005 John Wiley & Sons, Ltd

represent steps in the problem-solving process. One of the nodes is uniquely distinguished as the start or initial state, and there may be one or more nodes that represent the goal state or states. The task of a search algorithm is to find a solution path through the problem space, keeping track of the steps followed and states visited. Representing problems in computer science and bioinformatics as search problems allows the full weight of graph-theoretic concepts to be applied to the problem and also allows comparison between different solutions to the problem as well as comparisons between solutions to different problems.

3.2 Search algorithms

Consider the graph in Figure 3.1. Formally, a graph is collection of nodes (*vertices*) and links (*arcs*) connecting the nodes. In the example below the arcs are *labelled*, meaning that there is some cost to the link between two nodes. Usually these costs are distances when the graph represents a map, although such labels can also represent constraints to be satisfied before the link can be followed. For the moment we shall concentrate on graphs that represent maps, where if there is a label on an arc then it represents the distance between the two nodes it connects. If there is no label on an arc, the link shows that a path exists between the two nodes. The task in Figure 3.1 is to find the shortest route, in terms of distance and not cities visited, between S (the start city) and G (the goal city). There are eight 'cities' S, A, B, ..., G, but note that not all the cities are connected to each other. The distance between two nodes X and Y is the same as the distance between Y and X.

One possible solution route is S to A to D to G (SADG), giving a total distance of 18. Then SCDG may be noticed, with total distance 16, which

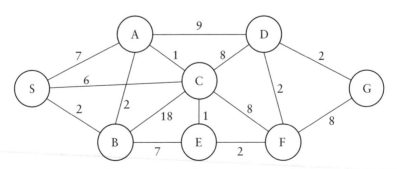

Figure 3.1   A graph representing a map

is shorter. After trying a number of possibilities, the route SBACEFDG may be arrived at, which gives a total distance of 12 even though all cities have been visited. To verify that this is indeed the shortest route, other routes have to be tried, but now there is a 'benchmark' of 12 which can be used to stop further examination of particular routes if the distance is 12 or more and G has not been reached.

The solution to this task is reached quickly, but now imagine that there is a real-life labelled map containing 100 or more cities and distances, with many different ways of getting from one city to another. A route may be found that appears the shortest, but how do we know for sure that it is the shortest? How long will it take to calculate the shortest route in such large-scale maps?

These may seem like hard questions to answer, so it may be decided to write programs to solve these problems. The first problem faced is how to represent the graph in Figure 3.1 to a computer. Fortunately, there is an easy way to represent graphs to computers which involves the *matrix* method (Table 3.1). Since matrices are provided as standard in most programming languages, there is an easy way to represent the connectivity of the graph in Figure 3.1. Providing the information to a computer in a way that the computer understands is to provide a *data structure* to the computer. Another advantage to the matrix method is that, if another node is added to the graph (another city is added to the map), it will be easy to add an extra row and column to the data structure and insert the distances between that node and all the nodes it connects to in the appropriate *x,y* entries, without needing to enter all the graph information again. Once such a data structure is developed, an *algorithm* is required that will make use of this data structure to calculate shortest routes.

An algorithm is a sequence of steps that, if systematically and correctly executed, will produce the desired result. For searching graphs there is a need to devise an algorithm that will explore paths rigorously, meaning that the solution is to be found as efficiently as possible as well as guaranteeing to return the correct result. To ensure that there is an efficient algorithm that doesn't explore a route that has been previously examined and found not to contain the desired solution, as well as exploring all possible routes that exist in the graph, a search algorithm is required that methodically searches routes one step at a time. The conventional way to do this is to convert the type of search into a *tree search*.

Look again at S, the start node (Figure 3.1). There are three links from S to A, B and C. Rather than decide arbitrarily to follow just one, all

Table 3.1   A matrix representation of the graph in Figure 3.1. Each city is numbered (S = 1, A = 2, etc). The rows of this distance or cost matrix describe the distance/cost between a start node and an end node, and the columns the distance/cost between an end node and a start node. For instance, row 1, column 4, contains the value 6. This entry states that there is distance 6 between S and C. Any distance can be accessed by giving (*x,y*) coordinates. For instance, (5,8) returns the value 2, which gives the distance between D and G. 'Ø' indicates that the two specified nodes are not connected. Note also that a node cannot be connected to itself (hence the Øs along the leading diagonal (1,1), (2,2) etc. of the matrix). Finally, note that the matrix is *symmetrical*. That is, the entries above the leading diagonal are the same as the entries below the leading diagonal, in mirror form. This reflects the property of the graph that the cost of getting from *x* to *y* is the same as the cost of getting from *y* to *x*. There may be graphs where this symmetry is not preserved (e.g. one-way streets between nodes which are shorter in one direction than the other)

	S 1	A 2	B 3	C 4	D 5	E 6	F 7	G 8
S 1	Ø	7	2	6	Ø	Ø	Ø	Ø
A 2	7	Ø	2	1	9	Ø	Ø	Ø
B 3	2	2	Ø	18	Ø	7	Ø	Ø
C 4	6	1	18	Ø	8	1	8	Ø
D 5	Ø	9	Ø	8	Ø	Ø	2	2
E 6	Ø	Ø	7	1	Ø	Ø	2	Ø
F 7	Ø	Ø	Ø	8	2	2	Ø	8
G 8	Ø	Ø	Ø	Ø	2	Ø	8	Ø

three are followed. This is represented in Figure 3.2(a). The start node is called the *root* of the tree and is at the top level. At the next level below are all the nodes (A, B, C) that can be reached from the start node. The tree at this stage is one level deep, and the tree at this point represents the routes SA, SB and SC. The nodes A, B and C are *child* nodes of S, and S is the *parent* node of A, B and C, which are *sibling* nodes to each other. Describing at a level below all the child nodes that can be reached from a parent node at the level above is called *expanding* the parent node. At the next level of the tree all the nodes that can be reached from A, B and C are then described (Figure 3.2(b)). A and B have three children nodes each, whereas C has five. The tree is now two levels deep and represents

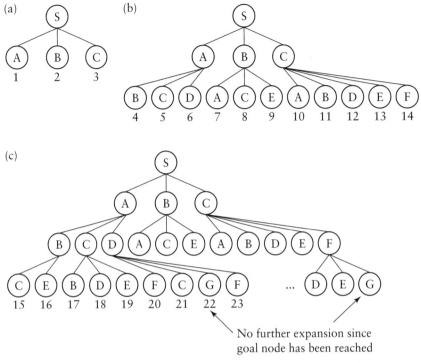

Figure 3.2   Ordered expansion of a search into a tree search

all the nodes that can be reached from S in two steps. For instance, the left-most path in Figure 3.2(b) describes the route SAB, whereas the right-most path the route SCF. It is ssumed that, when generating child nodes, there is no need to go back to the node which is its parent. The distance travelled each time the search is extended by a level can also be calculated, but another possibility is to generate all possible routes first without wasting time looking up distances in the matrix and then calculate the total distances of all paths at the end.

The next step in the expansion is given in Figure 3.2(c). Only a partial expansion of all nodes at the third level are described, but already it can be seen how complex the search tree is becoming. The search is continued until all paths reach G (all routes are *complete*), or it is not possible to expand a node without revisiting a node already visited earlier on the same path from the route node. Once the search stops, the distances for all paths can be calculated to identify the route with least cost (Figure 3.3).

To determine the number of paths that have been explored, they can be simply counted, as in the simple examples above. More generally, however, if a node has *b* child nodes, it is said to have a *branching*

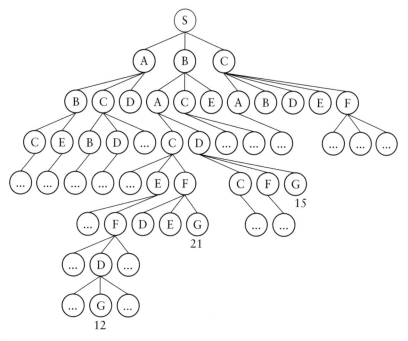

Figure 3.3   A fragment of the full breadth-first search tree is shown here (with dots in circles indicating that there are more sibling as well as child nodes that are not represented in the figure)

factor of *b*. If all paths are complete at the same level *d* of a tree and all nodes have *b* child nodes, then b^d will have been explored paths. For instance, if a tree had a branching factor of four (four child nodes from each expanded node) and all paths complete at level six, there will be 4^6 complete paths, i.e. 4096 complete paths. That is, at the first level there would be four child nodes to explore from the root node, i.e. 4^1 paths. At the next level, each of these four nodes would have had four child nodes themselves, giving 4^2 (i.e. 16) paths, and so on. The number of paths is pruned by preventing expansion of nodes to child nodes that had already been visited on the path, and for the example the number of child nodes for a parent was not fixed. If *on average* there are three child nodes from each expanded node, taking the pruning of redundant nodes into account, and the average depth of a complete path is six, even for the simple example above there would have been approximately 3^6 paths, i.e. 729 paths, to explore. However, imagine if there were a graph of 50 cities (for instance, a map of Great Britain), and each city could be connected to 10 other cities, and the average complete path depth was 25. That would give approximately 10^{25} paths, i.e. 10 000 000 000 000 000 000 000 000

(1 followed by 25 zeros) paths. Even if one billion paths per second could be processed on a truly fast computer, this would still take over 7.5 billion years to calculate. Generating all possible routes is clearly not feasible. Something a bit more intelligent is clearly needed, or the constraint needs to be loosened that the absolutely correct answer to the problem is required.

Breadth-first search

The technique for generating a search tree from a graph, as given in Figure 3.2, is *breadth-first*. Nodes are expanded in the order in which they are generated. For instance, in Figure 3.2, S is expanded into A, B and C, which are generated in the order 1, 2 and 3 (Figure 3.2(a)). Since A was first generated in the expansion of S, it is expanded first to B, C and D, which has generation order 4, 5 and 6; but before expanding any of these nodes, breadth-first searching goes back to node 2 (B) and expands that next to A, C and E (generation order 7, 8 and 9) and then goes back to node 3 and expands that to A, B, D, E and F (generation order 10, 11, 12, 13, 14). Nodes 1, 2 and 3 have therefore been expanded. Since node 4 (B) now comes first in terms of unexpanded nodes, it is expanded next, followed by node 5, etc.. If the task had been to find the route which visited fewest cities to get to G irrespective of distance, a breadth-first approach would have found the routes SADG, SCDG and SCFG at the third level (Figure 3.2(b)), and the search could have stopped at that point.

Depth-first search

The problem with a breadth-first search is in keeping a large number of routes in memory so that nodes can be expanded in the order generated, until all routes reach the destination node. Another technique for searching is *depth-first*, where the search tree is formed using the most recently generated node for further expansion (Figure 3.4).

Depth-first searching is advantageous when a solution is needed without caring about the number of nodes visited or the distance travelled. For instance, if only a route from S to G were required, it would have been found at node 13 (Figure 3.4) (in comparison with finding the shortest distance route at level 7 in Figure 3.3). Depth-first searches can also use less memory for storing paths. Each path can be explored until it reaches the goal node G, for instance, its distance calculated, and then

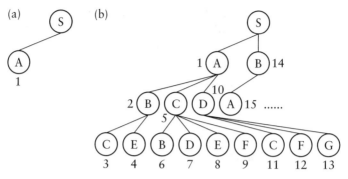

Figure 3.4 Depth-first search and expansion order

the path can be pruned with a record made of the distance for that route. However, depth-first searches must be supported by other checks that ensure that loops are not formed. For instance, if a large depth bound is set for the example graph in Figure 3.1, depth-first searching may loop around the path SABSABSAB. . .

3.3 Heuristic search methods

Depth-first and breadth-first searches are examples of 'blind' search techniques that systematically evaluate every path in the search space. However, when we humans search for a route from S to G in the map represented in Figure 3.1, we make choices of which paths to follow from a particular node depending on how much closer it gets to G. For instance, if we get to C from A, there does not seem much point in exploring the path to B because, in some sense, it takes the search backwards and not forwards in the search. Blind techniques, however, will explore the C to B path equally with others and may even explore this path ahead of the C to D or C to F if the algorithm requires nodes to be expanded, depth-first or breadth-first, in alphabetic order (as in Figures 3.2, 3.3 and 3.4, where child nodes are in alphabetic order). Once the algorithm is given some extra domain-specific information to help its search strategy, *heuristics* have been introduced.

A heuristic is any way that the algorithm can be directed towards solving the problem through the use of domain-specific information. That does not mean that the heuristic will always help solve the problem, but it may help the algorithm solve the problem more quickly than a blind approach. The main purpose is to reduce the search space by reducing the need to explore irrelevant or unlikely paths. A heuristic is therefore independent of an algorithm and can be described independently of that algorithm. For instance, a useful heuristic for the search of the graph in Figure 3.1 may be: 'When exploring paths, choose a path which takes the search closer to the goal.' The task then is to formalize this heuristic in a manner that is useful to the algorithm.

One way to formalize this heuristic is to give the algorithm some extra information in the form of an estimate of the *distance remaining* from a particular node to the goal node. This estimate is provided by the user and can be added to the data structure for the problem. For instance, as noted before, the matrix in Table 3.1 is semi-redundant in that, given that each path is bi-directional, the distance between node x and node y is the same as the distance between y and x. Also, since G is the goal, the last row of the matrix is redundant, since there is no need to leave G (generate paths beyond G). This last row can be replaced with a set of estimates concerning the distance remaining between all the other nodes and G (Table 3.2).

Table 3.2 The data structure for the graph in Figure 3.1, supplemented with estimates of the distance remaining in the final row. For instance, the second column value in the final row indicates that the estimated distance remaining between A and G is 20. These values can be estimated by, for instance, using information about the scale of the map represented by the graph in Figure 3.1. It is not important that these estimates are totally accurate

	S 1	A 2	B 3	C 4	D 5	E 6	F 7	G 8
S 1	Ø	7	2	6	Ø	Ø	Ø	Ø
A 2	7	Ø	2	1	9	Ø	Ø	Ø
B 3	2	2	Ø	18	Ø	7	Ø	Ø
C 4	6	1	18	Ø	8	1	8	Ø
D 5	Ø	9	Ø	8	Ø	Ø	2	2
E 6	Ø	Ø	7	1	Ø	Ø	2	Ø
F 7	Ø	Ø	Ø	8	2	2	Ø	8
G 8	30	20	25	15	5	18	5	Ø

Hill-climbing

When considering search problems such as this, the total number of solutions and their cost can be thought of as a landscape, with peaks and troughs representing collections of good and bad solutions. Most search problems have graduated peaks, which means that if the algorithm is at the bottom of a hill, then there is a set of steps to get to the top of that hill (see Figure 3.12 later in this chapter).

Simple hill-climbing, so called because of its drive towards better performing solutions, is a heuristically-informed search algorithm that expands a child node only if it is better than its parent node (Figure 3.5). Imagine the search starts with S and the task is to find a route to G. S is estimated to be 30 units of distance away from G (Table 3.2). The first child of S the algorithm explores is A. A is estimated to be 20 units of distance away from G. Since it is 'closer' to G than S, this node is selected. When A is reached, B (the first child, using alphabetical ordering) is examined. B is 25 units of distance away from G, which is further away than the estimated distance for A. So B is ignored for the moment. C, however, is estimated to be 15 units of distance away from G, which is a closer estimate than the 20 currently for A, so that path is followed. When C is reached, the path to B can be ignored since it appears to take the search further away from G according to the estimated distance remaining, but D appears to take the search closer (5 units of estimated distance remaining), so that path is taken. When D is reached, since going to A takes the search to a node already visited on the path, it is ignored. F is the same

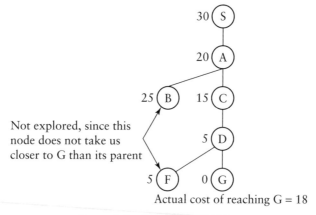

Not explored, since this node does not take us closer to G than its parent

Actual cost of reaching G = 18

Figure 3.5   Simple hill-climbing

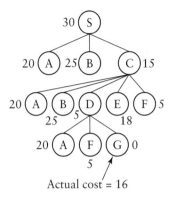

Actual cost = 16

Figure 3.6   Steepest-ascent hill-climbing with estimates of distance remaining

estimated distance away from G as D, so that can be ignored also. Then G is found, which is the goal node, so that path is taken.

However, the search is not over. One route to G with cost 18 has been found. The task is to find the shortest distance route, and other routes must be explored, especially those rejected earlier in the search due to estimated distances remaining that were larger than the parent node. However, at least there is now one path with an actual cost that can help guide the remainder of the search.

Steepest-ascent hill-climbing is a variation of hill-climbing that selects the best possible move at each point and requires all child nodes of a parent to be generated first before a decision is taken as to which child node to expand further (Figure 3.6). Again, even after the route SCDG is found, the search will need to explore the tree further to see if there are routes of shorter distance than 16.

Both depth-first and breadth-first searches expand only one node at a time. An extension to this is *beam search*, where two or more nodes are expanded in parallel with the other paths being kept in the background for subsequent checking, if required. The number of nodes explored in parallel is given by a *beam width*. An example of a heuristic beam search is given in Figure 3.7.

The search is started with S and its three child nodes. From the estimated distances remaining, two nodes A and C are chosen for further expansion at the next level. A has three child nodes and C has five. Three nodes all have estimated distance five remaining. Since two of these nodes are the same (D), one is chosen arbitrarily to expand further with F. At the third level, G is found twice, with different actual distances for the two different routes. Again, the beam search must return

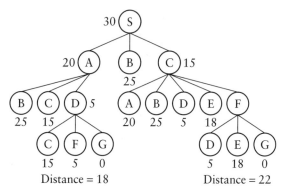

Figure 3.7   An example of a beam search with beam width two (that is, two nodes are expanded at each level)

to nodes not fully expanded to expand these further to see if a shorter route exists.

3.4 Optimal search strategies

While heuristic search methods using estimates of the distance remaining guide blind search techniques, it is clear that none of these techniques will find the route with the actual least distance SBACEFDG very easily, although such techniques can be useful for finding routes of shorter distance than previously known. For instance, if SCFG (distance 22) was previously used as a route, then finding SADG, while not the shortest route, leads to a better route than previously used. For certain applications it may be sufficient to find routes that are better than currently used ones, and heuristic search methods work well in these situations. However, if it is critically important to find the best or shortest route, *optimal search procedures* must be used. Optimal search procedures are distinguished from heuristic search methods by using the actual cost of the partial routes so far found in the search tree as a guide to which node to expand next. For instance, returning to the example in Figure 3.1, when S is expanded to A, C and B and there are three child nodes to expand next, an optimal search strategy would choose to expand B next because the actual cost of S to B, which is 2, is less than the actual cost of S to A (actual cost 7) and S to C (actual cost 6). After expanding B to A, C and E, the actual cost of S to B to A is 4, S to B to C is 20, and S to B to E is 9. Since S to B to A has least actual cost, it is chosen next. At some point, a route that is continually expanded will exceed the actual cost of another route elsewhere in the search tree, at which point a jump is made to whichever partial route has least actual cost so far.

Branch-and-bound and A*

This process of expanding (branching) nodes and then jumping to which ever route has least actual cost (binding to that route) is called *branch-and-bound* (or *best-first*) search. An example of branch-and-bound working on the example graph is given in Figures 3.8 and 3.9.

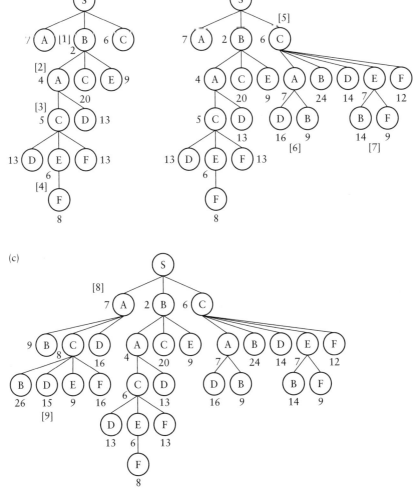

Figure 3.8 An example of branch-and-bound on the graph in Figure 3.1

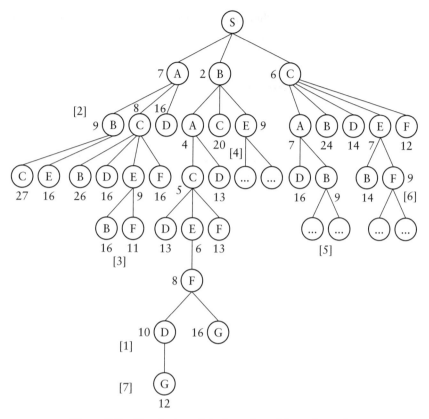

Figure 3.9   Conclusion of the branch-and-bound search

Actual costs of reaching a particular node on a route are given next to the node. The numbers in the diagram in square brackets refer to the order of the branch-and-bound search. In Figure 3.8(a), when S is expanded to A, B and C, the actual costs are used to determine which node to expand next, and since SB has lowest actual cost of 2, it is expanded first [1]. Since SBA has the lowest cost of 4 anywhere in the search tree, it is expanded next [2]. Since SBAC has the lowest cost of 5 anywhere in the tree, it is expanded further [3]. Since SBACE has joint lowest cost (with SC) of 6, and assuming it is chosen for expansion [4], the path SBACEF results (assuming that nodes already visited on the route are not revisited). At this point, SC has the lowest cost (Figure 3.8(b)), and the search now binds to SC [5]. After expansion of SC, SCA and SCE both have joint cost of 7, which is also the lowest anywhere in the search tree. After SCA [6] and SCE [7] are expanded, (c) SA has the lowest actual cost, so the search is now bound to that path (Figure 3.8(c)). SA is expanded to SAB, SAC and SAD [8], and SAC has the joint lowest cost with SBACEF. Assuming that SAC is expanded further [9], the lowest cost path anywhere in the tree is SBACEF (middle of tree).

The conclusion of the search is given in Figure 3.9. After SAC has been expanded (Figure 3.8(c)), the lowest actual cost partial route is SBACEF (with cost 8). This is expanded to D and G [1], and although G has been found with actual cost 15, the search must continue since there are many 'open' nodes that could still reach G with less cost. Since SAB now has the lowest route cost of 9 [2], this is expanded, as a result of which SACE [3] is expanded. This results in SBE having the lowest cost with 9, and so the search is bound there [4]. Assuming that the children nodes of SBE result in routes with a higher cost than 9, branching continues with SCAB [5], which has the lowest cost anywhere in the tree. Again assuming that the child nodes have greater cost, the search is then bound to SCEF [6], which also has cost 9. Finally, assuming that the child nodes of SCEF result in costs higher than 10 at some point, the search is bound back to SBACEFD [7], and the graph's true lowest cost path of 12 units of distance is found. However, all open nodes elsewhere in the tree on paths that have not yet resulted in a distance greater than 12 must be explored further until they reach G with less actual cost than 12, or their routes are greater than 12 and G has not been reached, at which point the search is terminated with SBACEFD returned as the real lowest-cost route.

While branch-and-bound is guaranteed to find the shortest (lowest-cost) route once all open nodes are explored to the point where there can be no more lowest-cost routes, there is still some efficiency to be gained by not keeping paths that reach a node with greater cost than another path in the search. For instance, in Figure 3.9 there is a path down the left side of the search tree that reaches C with cost 27 (SABC). Yet C is reached with one move from S with cost 6 at the first level (SC) of the search tree (on the right of the figure). There is no need to keep the higher cost path SABC since C is already reached with lower cost. SABC can therefore be pruned in Figure 3.9. Applying a similar line of reasoning, SAC (cost 8) and SBC (cost 20) should have been pruned, leaving the search with fewer paths to explore. An efficiency principle here is that if two or more paths reach a common node then only the path that reaches the common node with minimum cost should be kept and the rest deleted. Also, just as hill-climbing benefited from the inclusion of heuristic information as to whether the search was heading in the right direction, some distance-remaining estimates can be used to guide the search. The result is the A* algorithm, which is a branch-and-bound search supplemented by the deletion of redundant paths and the use of estimates of distance remaining. Figures 3.10 and 3.11 show how the graph in Figure 3.1 would be searched by A*, using the distance remaining estimates contained in Table 3.2.

After expanding S (Figure 3.10(a)) each node is given an '*x/y*' pair of values, where '*x*' is the estimated distance remaining plus actual cost, and '*y*' is the actual cost only. The node with the least '*x*' value is expanded first [1]. This results in five child nodes [2]. Since there is an alternative path to A with less or equal cost elsewhere in the search tree (SA has cost 7; SCA also has cost 7), one is pruned (in this case SCA). Similarly, SCB can also be pruned since there is a path with less cost to B elsewhere in the search tree (SB). There are two least '*x*' values of 19 (SCD and SCF), and imagine that SCD is expanded first (Figure 3.10(b)) through some form of random tie-break [3]. Two child nodes can be pruned, since there are less actual cost paths to these nodes elsewhere (SCDA (actual cost 23) can be pruned because of SA (actual cost 7), and SCDF (16) because of SCF (14). Also, the first route to G with actual cost 16 is found (SCDG), which acts as a benchmark or threshold for the subsequent search. The search must continue (Figure 3.10(c)) since there are several open paths still left to explore. SCF is expanded because its '*x*' value is lowest of anywhere in the search tree. All three child nodes can be pruned [4] since there are less actual distance paths to these nodes elsewhere. Since all child nodes of F have been checked, it too can be pruned. Since SCE has the lowest '*x*' value, it is expanded (Figure 3.10(d)). The path to B can be pruned [5], F is expanded (least cost '*x*' value), the route to G is pruned since there is an actual less-cost path elsewhere to G [6], and D is expanded because of its '*x*' value of 15. The path to A is pruned [7], and a new, actual lower-cost route to G is found (actual cost 13). The previous best route to G (SCDG) can now be pruned [8].

The second and final part of the search is provided in Figure 3.11. The lowest '*x*' value for an open node is SA (assuming a random tie-break with SB, Figure 3.11(a)). All three child nodes can be reached with less actual cost elsewhere in the search tree, and so A and its child nodes can be pruned [9]. SB is expanded (Figure 3.11(b)) with two child nodes pruned [10]. SBA is expanded and one of its child nodes is pruned [11]. SBAC is kept because it reaches C with less actual cost (5) than SC (6) . SBAC is expanded, and two child nodes are pruned [12]. SBACE is expanded [13] and F kept since this is the least actual cost way of reaching F. One of its two child nodes is deleted [14], since there is an actual less-cost

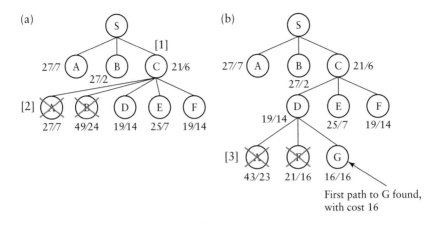

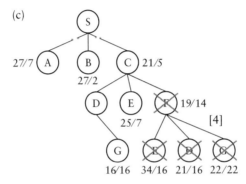

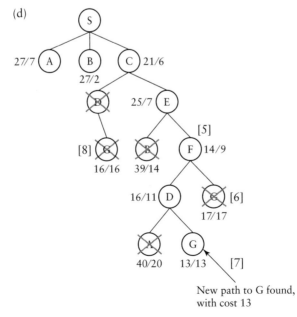

Figure 3.10 The first half of A* searching the example graph

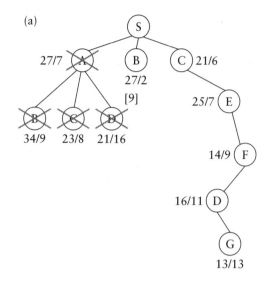

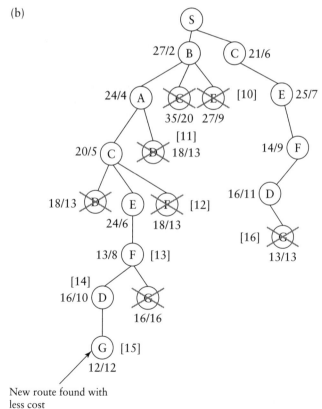

New route found with
less cost

Figure 3.11 The final part of A* search

way of reaching G, and finally G is found [15]. Since SBACEGDG is less actual cost than the previously found route to G (SCEFDG), the latter is pruned [16]. Since there are no more open nodes to examine, A* has found the shortest (least actual cost) route from S to G.

3.5 Problems with search techniques

There are three major problems with any search technique that uses some distance remaining metric: *foothills*, *plateaux* and *ridges*. Foothills are *local maxima* that deflect the search to areas that initially look promising but on further investigation turn out not to lead to the goal (Figure 3.12(a)). All moves from the top of the search hill look worse than an earlier position. Apart from wasting time and resource, there is the problem of how to redirect the search in the most appropriate direction. Plateaux occur when the distance remaining values for child nodes are

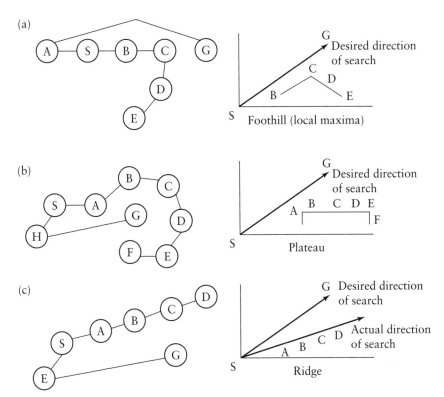

Figure 3.12   Problems with search techniques using the distance remaining; S is the start node and G the goal node

identical or nearly identical (Figure 3.12(b)). No obvious route can be found to the goal. Ridges occur when the search appears to be heading in the right direction, but the further one goes the more distant the goal actually becomes (Figure 3.12(c)). Some methods for dealing with these problems are: to backtrack (i.e. systematically work back through the route to identify the point where the problem started and resume search by expanding an alternative node), to jump randomly anywhere in the search tree and to explore an expansion several moves ahead to see if that route looks promising before committing the search to it.

3.6 Complexity of search

The example graph contained in Figure 3.1 is deliberately designed to show how complex a search can be without heuristic knowledge. A total of 34 paths were examined in Figure 3.10 and Figure 3.11 before the optimal path was found. Given an average branching factor b of three and an average depth of route d to G of five, the figure of 34 is to be compared with a figure of $b^d = 3^5 = 243$ paths that might have had to be explored exhaustively if A* had not been used or information gathered earlier in the search to guide subsequent search. Nevertheless, the graph might be such that it is necessary to explore all possible paths before finding the shortest route. The *time complexity* of A*, in the worst case, is $O(b^d)$, where 'O' stands for 'of the order of'. This notation helps to identify the amount of time A* might actually take to identify the shortest route in the worst case. If 100 paths can be explored every second, then $O(b^d)$ for the graph in Figure 3.1, given $b = 3$ and $d = 5$, is 2.43 s. If the branching factor had been greater, say, $b = 4$ or $b = 5$, then the amount of time would be 10.24 s ($4^5 = 1024$ paths) and 31.25 s ($5^5 = 3125$ paths), respectively. If, however, the branching factor remains constant and the depth of the tree increases to $d = 6$ or $d = 7$ (that is, the best route is on average 6 or 7 levels down the search tree), then A* would take, in the worst case, 7.29 s ($3^6 = 729$ paths) and 21.87 s ($3^7 = 2187$ paths). The O notation here helps estimate how long a search will take in the worst possible case.

It may be asked what the 'worst possible case' means here. Consider a depth-first search, with the search tree expanding the most recently generated nodes first (Figure 3.4), where the desired shortest path is on the extreme right-hand side of the search tree. A depth-first search would then need to generate every possible route to find the best route, and this is the worst possible case. A depth-first search is therefore also $O(b^d)$

(assuming some form of backtracking so that nodes generated earlier in the search tree are revisited to be expanded later in the search tree). Sometimes the shortest route might be on the very left of the tree, and its structure is such that all remaining routes can be pruned immediately without any need to expand them further. In this 'best possible case' the solution has been found in $O(d)$, that is, within the time it takes to generate a route of average length. The O notation is not meant to take into account practical aspects of computation, such as processor speed, but is meant to give an abstract description in terms of units of time, however measured, of how long an algorithm will take to complete its task, in the worst possible case.

The 'O' notation is also used to estimate space requirements for a search. For instance, with A*, in the worst case, all paths found in the search tree may need to be stored because the shortest route is not found until the very end of the search and no pruning of redundant paths is possible. The space complexity of this worst-case scenario is also $O(b^d)$. For instance, if it takes 1 byte to store a node and its path to a child, then for A*, with $b = 3$ and $d = 5$, 243 bytes are needed. For a search with $b = 10$ and $d = 10$, 10 billion bytes would be needed.

It is better, from a computational complexity viewpoint, to have algorithms that are of the order $O(x^k)$, where x can vary and k is a constant number, than to have an algorithm of the order $O(k^x)$. Consider algorithms of the order $O(1^2)$, $O(2^2)$, $O(3^2)$, $O(4^2)$, $O(5^2)$, etc., i.e. $O(x^k)$. The values are $O(1)$, $O(4)$, $O(9)$, $O(16)$, $O(15)$, etc. Compare this to algorithms of the order $O(2^1)$, $O(2^2)$, $O(2^3)$, $O(2^4)$, $O(2^5)$, etc., i.e. $O(k^x)$. The values here are $O(2)$, $O(4)$, $O(8)$, $O(16)$, $O(32)$, etc. In the latter case, there is an *exponential* increase in the complexity (the exponent of k^x increases), whereas in the former there is a *polynomial* increase (the polynomial of x^k increases).

With regard to an $O(b^d)$ search, it is better to have the branching factor b increase than the depth d of the tree increase. For instance, consider an algorithm of $O(70^2)$, that is, each node has 70 connections (with 70 or more nodes) but the best route can be found at level 2 of the search tree. This results in 4900 paths to explore. On the other hand, if there were just two connections from each node, the best route will be found at level 70, i.e. $O(2^{70})$. This might happen with a 70 city map where each node was connected to just two other nodes. The task of finding the shortest route that visits every city would now mean that the resulting number of paths is too large for any computer to calculate. In fact, it is estimated that there are about 2^{70} atoms in the whole universe. Even assuming one atom per path, all the atoms in the universe would be required just to store all the paths if a depth-first search or A* is used. Unfortunately, most of the really interesting problems, including several in bioinformatics, have search spaces and algorithms which are exponential in nature. Also, no attempt has been made to assess the cost of actually running the algorithm in the above cases, and this cost must also be included in the estimates of how long an algorithm will take to find the right solution.

3.7 Use of graphs in bioinformatics

The graph in Figure 3.1 provided an example of maps that can be searched for routes. Such graphs can also be used to check whether specific routes exist between two nodes. For example, if it is asked whether a route exists that starts from S and visits only cities A and F on the way to G, no such route exists. After A, another city has to be visited to reach F. In other words, the sequence SAFG is not a route of the map, whereas SADFG is. Another sequence SDFG is also not a valid route of the map. Graphs can therefore be used not just to generate routes but also to check potential routes or, in this case, the sequence of cities that must be visited between the start and end nodes. Such a sequence can be regarded as a string of characters, and the task is to determine whether the string is a valid string, or sequence of characters, according to the structure and content of an *automaton*.

Consider the problem of constructing a graph that accepts the following four DNA sequences as valid:

ACAATG
ACAAATC
AGAATC
ACCGATC

Figure 3.13 contains a special sort of graph, called an automaton, that shows how these four sequences can be 'accepted' by the automaton. An automaton adds direction to the arcs in the graph which specify the way in which links must be followed. This automaton consists of labelled states 1 to 8, with directed connections between these states. State 1 is the start state, and states 7 and 8 the final state. Each directed connection is labelled with a letter which specifies that the connection can only be followed if the letter is encountered as the next symbol in the string. For instance, to accept ACAATG, start in state 1 and follow the link to 2, since the label A on the arc going out from 1 is encountered as the first character of the sequence. In the act of following a link, the move is

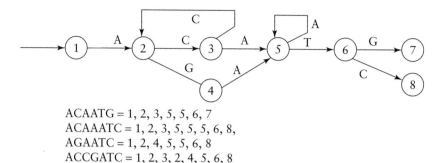

ACAATG = 1, 2, 3, 5, 5, 6, 7
ACAAATC = 1, 2, 3, 5, 5, 5, 6, 8,
AGAATC = 1, 2, 4, 5, 5, 6, 8
ACCGATC = 1, 2, 3, 2, 4, 5, 6, 8

Figure 3.13 A graph as automaton

made to the next character of the sequence (C). In state 2, there are two choices, and the link to state 3 is followed since the current character is C. The next character is A, and so on. The numbers by the four sequences at the bottom left of the diagram provide a history (trace) of the states entered. If a character is encountered that does not permit the exit from a state that is not a final state, the automaton 'stops' and a reject answer is returned, i.e. the sequence is not accepted by the automaton. Only if the automaton stops in a final state (there are no more characters to be processed) is the sequence accepted. Notice that loops back to earlier states and self-states are allowed.

A matrix representation can still be used to represent the graph as automaton, as provided in Table 3.3. The entries in the table are not distances but *conditions* that must be satisfied if there is to be a transition from one node (state) to another. Such conditions become the characters that must exist in specific positions of the sequence if the sequence as a whole is to be accepted as valid.

Expressions and grammar

An *expression* can be derived that provides a general description of the structure of any sequence that will be accepted by this automaton if some extra notation is added to the sequence. Let '*' mean 'zero or more occurrences', '+' mean 'one or more occurrences', and '[|]' mean 'or', with the alternatives provided on either side of the middle stick. Then the four sequences ACAATG, ACAAATC, AGAATC and ACCGATC can be expressed as 'A [G | C+ | C+G] A* T [G | C]'. That is, a sequence is accepted by this automaton if (i) it starts with an A, followed by (ii) G, or by one or more occurrences of C ('C+'), or by one or more Cs followed by a G ('C+G'), followed by (iii) zero or more As ('A*'), followed by

Table 3.3   Two ways of representing the automaton in Figure 3.13. In the top table, a blank entry means that no path exists between the node number given in the row and the node number given in the column. A transition between two nodes is permitted only if the character given in the appropriate cell is encountered. Otherwise, the automaton stops and 'rejects' the string. If the automaton stops in state 7 or state 8, this means that the string is accepted. In the bottom table, each entry in the table specifies which state the automaton is to switch to if a character is encountered in a particular state, as given by the row. For instance, if the automaton is in state 1 (row labelled 1) and an 'A' is encountered, then the automaton switches to state 2. A blank entry means that no transition is possible and the automaton therefore cannot proceed. The entries in boldface (row 6) specify the terminal (accept) states.

	1	2	3	4	5	6	7	8
1 = start node		A						
2			C	G				
3		C			A			
4					A			
5					A	T		
6							G	C
7 = goal node								
8 = goal node								

	A	C	G	T
1	2			
2		3	4	
3	5	2		
4	5			
5	5			6
6		8	7	

(iv) one T, followed by (v) either a G or a C. The state numbers in the automaton are useful for converting this complex expression into six transition rules, as follows:

1   sequence → A S2

2   S2 → C S3 | G S4

3   S3 → C S2 | A S5

4   S4 → A S5

5   S5 → A S5 | T S6

6   S6 → G | C

That is, a sequence starts with an 'A' followed by state 2 ('**S2**'), according to rule (1). State 2 is either a 'C' followed by **S3** or a 'G' followed by **S4**, according to rule (2), and so on. Boldface is used to distinguish the states of the automaton from the characters of the string. The special start symbol **sequence** is used to signify that the set of rules (1) to (6) starts with rule (1). Such a set of rules, together with a specification of the symbols that are allowed, including notation symbols such as '→' and '|' as well as a special start symbol, is called a *grammar*. A trace of how, for instance, the first of the sequences above has been generated with this grammar, is as follows:

sequence → A **S2** → AC **S4** → ACA **S5** → ACAA **S5** → ACAAT **S6** → ACAATG

The grammar (1) – (6) above contains two types of symbols, apart from the rewrite ('→') and alternative ('|') symbols. The symbols in boldface are *non-terminals*, meaning that they are symbols that appear on the left-hand side of rules for expansion and also on the right-hand side of some rules to allow for loops. The symbols not in boldface are *terminal* symbols, meaning that such symbols cannot be expanded further and are actual characters of the sequence.

When a grammar contains rules of the form **S** → X or **S** → X **Y** only, that is, when the right-hand side of all rules of a grammar contain either only one terminal symbol X or a terminal symbol X followed at most by one non-terminal **Y**, this is a *a right-linear regular grammar*. Sequence expressions that attempt to describe strings accepted or generated by such grammars, such as the expression 'A [G | C$^+$ | C$^+$G] A* T [G | C]', are called *regular expressions*. Such grammars are among the simplest grammars possible, and it is easy to construct *finite-state automata*, such as the one provided in Figure 3.13, for the sequences either generated or accepted by such grammars. For every regular expression or regular grammar, there is an equivalent finite-state automaton that represents or describes it, and vice versa. Regular expressions are used widely in bioinformatics to search for sequences matching a particular pattern, as given by the regular expression, in DNA or protein sequence databases. When a regular expression is input to the database, a finite state automaton is generated from the regular expression that efficiently and speedily scans the DNA or protein sequences in the database to identify partial and total matches against the expression.

3.8 Grammars, languages and automata

Grammars and automata can be used to study the types of problem that can be solved with a computer. A grammar is formally defined to consist of an *alphabet*, combinations of symbols from this alphabet to form *strings*, and a *language* that contains all the permissible strings according to the *rules* of the grammar. More precisely, an alphabet for DNA, for example, consists of the four symbols 'A', 'C', 'G' and 'T', and this is formally specified using '$\sum$' (capital sigma): $\sum = \{A,C,G,T\}$.

A string is any random combination of these symbols, such as 'AAAAA', 'ACGTACGTACGT' and 'GGGGCCCCTTTTAAAA'. The task of a grammar is to specify which of these strings is acceptable or valid according to the rules of the grammar. For instance, in the previous use of graphs to represent maps, any random combination of city sequences (e.g. 'SAASAGSA') can be generated, but only a small number of those combinations are valid according to the actual graph (Figure 3.1). The graph therefore expresses the permitted combinations of city sequences ('SADG' is a valid sequence or route whereas 'SDAG' is not). The task of a grammar, or graph as automaton, is therefore to identify the subset of random combinations of symbols (strings) that are actually permitted. For instance, the graph in Figure 3.1 can be represented as a grammar (without concern about the distances):

(i)   S → SA | SB | SC

(ii)   A → AS | AB | AC | AD

(iii) B → BS | BA | BC | BE

(iv)   C → CS | CA | CB | CD | CE | CF

(v)   D → DA | DC | DE | DF | DG

(vi)   E → EB | EC | EF

(vii) F → FC | FD | FE | FG

(viii) G → G

Note the difference between boldface symbols and non-boldface symbols. For instance, rule (i) states that the non-terminal S can be rewritten or transformed into terminal S followed by non-terminal B or non-terminal C or non-terminal D. These eight rules of the grammar all have a non-terminal on the left-hand side of the rule and a terminal followed by a non-terminal symbol on the right-hand side of the rule (i.e. the rules are right linear). Notice also that the only way to 'exit' the rules is at some point to rewrite G as G only (rule (viii)). The alphabet for this grammar is therefore $\sum = \{S,A,B,C,D,E,F,G,S,A,B,C,D,E,F,G\}$ and valid strings (routes) of the grammar are, for example:

(a) $S \rightarrow SA \rightarrow SAD \rightarrow SADF \rightarrow SADFG \rightarrow SADFG$

(b) $S \rightarrow SC \rightarrow SCS \rightarrow SCSC \rightarrow SCSCF \rightarrow SCSCFG \rightarrow SCSCFG$

That is, of all the possible random combinations of the letters S to G, only those combinations starting with S and ending with G where the letters in-between are sequenced according the rules constitute the *language* accepted by the graph as automaton. Some of these combinations will contain loops, such as in the second derivation (b) above where the route revisits S from C, which in terms of routes may not be desirable. If that is the case, directions (arrows) will need to be put on the links between the cities to prevent such loops and the grammar rewritten accordingly.

Automata theory

In *automata theory* the task is usually to determine whether strings are part of the language according to the rules of the grammar and using the symbols of the alphabet. One of the significant discoveries in computer science was the realization that this formulation of automata theory was general enough to cover all computational problems. For instance, even asking for the product of two numbers m and n is equivalent to asking which one of the strings '$m \times n = 1$', '$m \times n = 2$', '$m \times n = 3$', '$m \times n = 4$', '$m \times n = 5$', '$m \times n = 6$', etc., is valid according to the rules of grammar called 'arithmetic', where m and n are non-terminals that can be rewritten in a variety of ways (e.g. $m \rightarrow 1|2|3|4|\ldots$). For instance, '$2 \times 3 = 6$' is a valid string whereas '$2 \times 3 = 5$' is not.

Finite-state automata are not adequate for coping with certain nested structures found in biosequences, however. RNA sequences sometimes contain loops, whereby the RNA folds back on itself to form a double strand (Figure 3.14). RNA can form a looped structure when there is complementary base pairing within a sequence. In the left-hand figure, the mRNA primary sequence 'NNNNNAAAAAAAAAAAUUUUUUUU-UUNNNNN', where 'N' stands for any nucleotide, forms a secondary structure loop when the subsequence 'AAAAAAAAAAUUUUUUUUUU'

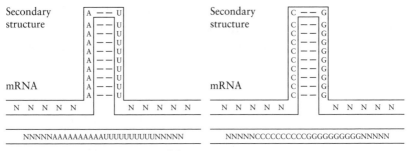

Figure 3.14   Looped RNA structure with equal numbers of complementary base

pairs with its complement bases, and similarly for the right-hand figure involving Cs and Gs. Such looping can form the basis for removing introns from mRNA, where the loop is 'cut' out and the sequence 'NNNNNNNNN' is left as the exon. Also, non-translated transcripts for transfer RNA (tRNA) can form such loops, called 'hairpins', which are required for the correct functioning of tRNA.

To cope with arbitrary long expressions where there is a specific relationship between two or more symbols, a more powerful grammar than a regular grammar is needed. For instance, here is a way of capturing the information that only those sequences that contain an equal amount of two symbols are strings of the language as follows: $L = \{A^nU^n \,|\, C^nG^n, n \geq 1\}$. That is, a valid string of the language is some number n of As followed by the same number of Us, or some number n of Cs followed by the same number of Gs, where n is greater than or equal to 1. In grammar terms, the rules for such structures can be:

loop → loop₁| loop₂
loop₁→ AU | A loop₁U
loop₂→ CG | C loop₂ G

The *recursion* of loop₁ and loop₂ (that is, the occurrence of loop₁ and loop₂ on both the left-hand and right-hand side of their rules) allows for loop₁ or loop₂ to be incorporated as many times as one needs. An example of a trace is: loop → loop₂ → *C* loop₂*G* → C*C* loop₂*G*G → CC*C* loop₂*G*GG → CCCCGGGG, where italics signify the most recently inserted nucleotides. The recursion terminates when loop₁ or loop₂ is expanded without either recurring, as in the final step of the trace above.

The automaton in Figure 3.15(a) is a finite-state automaton that is not powerful enough, since it accepts strings where there are an unequal number of complementary characters. Given the grammar for generating

(a) Finite state automaton

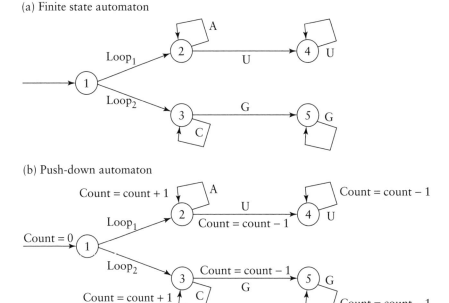

(b) Push-down automaton

Figure 3.15   The difference between a finite-state automaton and a push-down automaton

loops (Figure 3.13), a finite-state automaton (FSA) will not be powerful enough to accept only those strings specified by the grammar. That is, while the FSA will accept strings of the form 'AAAUUU' and 'CCCGGG' it will also accept, incorrectly, strings of the form 'AUUU' and 'CCCCG'. In other words, an FSA has no memory of what has occurred earlier in the string but simply moves from state to state depending on the symbol encountered in the input string. It is possible (Figure 3.15(a)), however, to construct a *push-down automaton* (PDA) by attaching some memory to the automaton in the form of a count variable which is incremented every time the symbol 'A' or 'C' is encountered and decremented every time the symbol 'U' or 'G' is encountered. If it is stipulated that that only those strings that result in the PDA terminating in states 4 and 5 with count equal to zero are accepted, then only those strings that have an equal number of As followed by an equal number of Us (and equal number of Cs followed by an equal number of Gs) will indeed be accepted. The PDA is 'more powerful' than the FSA in that it accepts fewer strings than the FSA.

A 'more powerful' grammar or automaton results in *fewer* strings being accepted (or generated) than a finite state automaton. 'More powerful', in computational terms, means satisfying more constraints. That is, a finite state automaton can accept or generate strings of the form X^nY^m (any number of Xs followed by any number of Ys), some of which will satisfy the constraint that $n = m$ by chance (for instance, three Xs followed by three Ys). However, once it is decided to accept only a subset of these strings, namely, only those strings where there is a specified relationship between the number of Xs and the number of Ys, a more powerful formalism and automaton are required. Also, the type of information that can appear on a link has been increased to include an action, whereas a finite-state automaton can only have conditions. In this case, the action consists of updating a counter which must be stored in memory. Therefore, a push-down automaton requires a memory, and that is what makes the automaton able to deal with strings where there are constraints concerning the number of occurrences of two symbols in the string.

More powerful automata

Imagine that the task now is to accept or generate strings where there is a dependency between three symbols in a string, such as an equal number of Xs, Ys and Zs, in that order. For example, the language may be: $L = \{A^nC^n U^n, n \geq 1\}$. A push-down automaton will now not be powerful enough. If only one counter variable is used to check that the number of Xs is equal to the number of Ys, when the counter returns to zero after the last Y there will be no information as to how many Xs and Ys were encountered. What is required is a second counter which is set to the same value as the number of Xs first encountered, so that it stores this information even after the first counter is returned to 0 after the last Y. An automaton with two memory counters is called a *linear-bounded automaton* (LBA, Figure 3.16). An LBA is required to accept strings where there are specified relationships between three symbols.

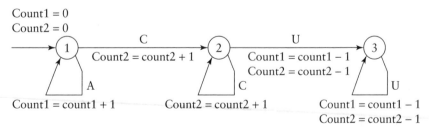

Figure 3.16   A linear-bounded automaton (LBA)

Two counter variables are now required to accept only those strings that conform to $L = \{A^n\ C^n\ U^n, n \geq 1\}$, that is, only strings containing one or more As followed by the same number of Cs followed by the same number of Us. The first counter counts the number of As and the second the number of Cs. Both counters are decremented with every U found. Any string that does not finish in state 3 with count1 and count2 equal to zero is rejected by this LBA.

If there is a need to check for relationships between more than three symbols in a string, a *Turing Machine* – which essentially has an infinite number of counters available – is required. Turing Machines are the most powerful type of computing machine imaginable. That is, while no real Turing Machines exist (because of the need for an infinite number of counters or, as is more conventionally stated, an infinite memory) there is no more powerful machine imaginable, if by 'machine' is meant some mechanism that can follow an algorithm systematically and rigorously to return a correct result. Bioinformatics has fortunately so far not required the use of an automaton that is the equivalent of a Turing Machine for solving problems in biology.

One of the reasons for looking at the relationship between languages, grammars and automata in some detail is to relate the types of problem that can be computed with classes of *complexity*. A finite-state automaton solves problem in *linear* time. For instance, if it takes the finite-state automaton in Figure 3.13 five units of time to process the string ACATG (one unit of time for each symbol), then it will take 10 units of time to process ACAAAAATG (one unit of time for each path followed). This is because the rules of a regular grammar only allow the occurrence of one terminal symbol or, if a non-terminal symbol appears, only one non-terminal which in turn can be expanded only as one terminal symbol. A push-down automaton for accepting strings of a context-free language will take longer than linear time, since any combination of symbols can appear on the right-hand side of a rule. This increases the branching factor of the tree used to generate sequences which, as seen earlier with regard to search trees, leads to *polynomial* time increase, where the increase depends on the number of branches possible at each node of the tree. After push-down automata, complexity becomes at least *exponential* (the depth of the tree increases) and, in the case of a Turing Machine, *semi-decidable*. That is, if there is a problem that requires the power of a Turing Machine, it has to be accepted that the automaton may loop forever for some strings which are not strings of the language. The automaton will keep trying different ways to identify whether the string is or is not a string of the language. If the string is indeed a string of the language, the Turing Machine will eventually stop in an accept state. If, however, the string is not a string of the language, it is possible that the Turing Machine will not stop in a reject state. It may loop forever trying to find a way of accepting the string. It will not be known when to switch off the automaton, since we it will not be known if the Turing Machine will loop forever or would have found the answer (which may be an accept) the moment after the automaton is switched off. For most strings that are not part of the language the Turing Machine will eventually halt in a reject state, but one of the most important findings in computer science is that it is not possible to predict for which non-strings the Turing Machine will halt in a reject state and for which strings it will loop forever (the halting problem). That is, it is not possible to find or run an algorithm that, prior to running the Turing Machine with that algorithm on some sequence, will decide in all cases whether that Turing Machine will halt or not for that sequence.

3.9 Classes of problems

This leads to a classification of problems that are P (for polynomial), NP (for *non-deterministic* polynomial), and *NP-complete*. A problem falls in the class P if it can be solved at worst in polynomial time (such as with a push-down automaton). A problem falls in the class NP if it can only be solved by a Turing Machine that allows more than one branch with the same label. However, since there are a number of possible exit routes from a node in the automaton for the same character in the string, all of them will need to be tried. Since a Turing Machine can do what it likes with the string, including rewriting it, it will not be known when to stop the machine if it continues to run for a long time. All that can be said is that, if the string is a valid string of the language, the Turing Machine will eventually halt. The reason this class of problems is called non-deterministic *polynomial* is to express the theoretical view that, if there is an infinite number of machines each of which could explore each path of the search tree in parallel, the problem could be solved in polynomial time. However, some problems are such that the exponential nature of the problem may soon lead to there being more paths to explore than computers on the planet, or even the universe. Finally, the class *NP-complete* refers to those problems that are NP but where the solution, if returned, can be verified in linear or polynomial time at worst. For instance, searching for any route between S and G is an exponential problem, but when a route is found it can be verified by simply following the route and seeing if the route starts at S and finishes at G (i.e. linear time depending on the number of cities visited). However, to verify a shortest route returned by the search algorithm can take as long as searching the tree to start off with. That is, a check needs to be made that among all the other routes there is no shorter route. One of the biggest unsolved problems in computer science is to determine whether, for all the problems that fall in the class *NP* (but not for the class *NP-complete*), there are algorithms that have not yet been found for solving these problems in polynomial time, i.e. does *NP* = *P*? There are theoretical findings that indicate that, if a polynomial-time solution can be found for just one of the problems in the *NP* class, there will be polynomial-time solutions for all problems in the *NP* class. However, so far no one has managed to conclusively prove that a single problem in *NP* actually falls in the class *P*.

These comments on complexity assume that what is required is always to find the provably best or optimal answer to a problem. For instance, the problem of finding the provably best alignment in a multiple sequence alignment problem is an *NP* problem (there are many different locations to insert gaps, for instance), but often a good solution is required rather than the best solution. Also, the complexity of an algorithm for solving a problem always assumes a worst-case scenario, which will sometimes but not always occur. Great savings in time can also be obtained if solutions are required that are better than those currently available (heuristic solutions), or solutions which are as close to optimal as can be determined within a specified bound (approximated solutions).

This chapter has shown that, while new technology allows researchers to compute solutions to ever more complex problems, some tasks can require more computation than is possible with every computer running for the rest of time. Even some apparently simple tasks such as finding the shortest path through a graph, or searching for matching strings, can be *NP*-complete. Therefore for many problems in science, engineering and, most importantly, bioinformatics, more intelligent search and optimization strategies must be used. The heuristic hill-climbing methods seen in this chapter are among the simplest of the search methods covered in this book. These first three chapters have laid the foundations of biology, bioinformatics and computer science. The remainder of the book describes the many intelligent methods currently in use in bioinformatics, ranging from the commonly-used standard methods to the more unusual and yet-to-be applied techniques.

3.10 Summary of chapter

1   Graphs consist of nodes (vertices) connected by links (arcs). Many problems in computer science and bioinformatics can be converted into a graph form for search purposes.

2   Searching graphs can be through exhaustive or heuristic methods. Exhaustive methods typically use depth-first or breadth-first methods to search the tree systematically. Heuristic methods require some domain-specific information, such as distance remaining estimates, to guide the search.

3   Hill-climbing is a popular heuristic method for a search. Simple hill-climbing takes the first option that is better than where the search currently is, whereas steepest-ascent hill-climbing examines all child nodes first before choosing the best path.

4   Hill-climbing does not guarantee to find the optimal path. Branch-and-bound methods, supplemented by pruning of redundant nodes and the distance remaining, do guarantee to find the optimal path.

5   In all search cases, the complexity of the search increases as the number of nodes and links increases. This can be problematic for a number of bioinformatics problems requiring a search, such as accepting or generating strings of characters.

6   Finite-state automata are a method for dealing with regular grammars and the expressions generated by such grammars. They are efficient but lack the power to deal with strings where there is some relationship between two or more symbols in strings.

7   Push-down automata can handle strings in which there is some relationship between two symbols but need some memory to work effectively. Some bioinformatics phenomena, such as looped RNA structures, require the power of a push-down automaton. Languages handled by push-down automata require context-free grammars for their generation.

8   Beyond context-free grammars lies increased complexity (linear-bounded automata and Turing Machines). Problems can be classified

as polynomial or non-deterministic polynomial. Polynomial problems require polynomial algorithms that grow linearly in terms of memory and time or at worst they grow in polynomial time. Non-deterministic polynomial (NP) problems are characterized by exponential growth. Unfortunately, a number of problems in bioinformatics fall in the NP class.

3.11 Further reading

Hopcroft, J.E., Motwani, R. and Ullman, J.D. (2000) *Introduction to Automata Theory, Languages and Computability*, 2nd edn, Addison Wesley.

Luger, G.F. (2002) *Artificial Intelligence: Structures and Strategies for Complex Problem Solving*, Addison Wesley.

Winston, P.H. (1992) *Artificial Intelligence*. Addison Wesley.

Part 2
Current Techniques

4
Probabilistic Approaches

4.1 Introduction to probability

Probability is the branch of mathematics which is concerned with the likelihood that events will occur. It is an invaluable tool for scientists since an event is often not guaranteed to occur, but can only be characterized by the fact that it will occur an average number of times given a number of trials. This is also of particular importance to bioinformaticians as the interactions and reactions that occur in biological processes can often only be characterized by probability theory. Probability theory can also be useful in determining the underlying structure of datasets or sequences. This chapter firstly provides a short background to probability and then details a number of the probabilistic approaches to bioinformatics problems.

Conditional probability is different from *frequentist* probability. For example, if 55 per cent of the students in a department are female and 45 per cent are male, then the event: 'a randomly selected student is female' has a probability, according to the frequentist approach, of 0.55, where the probability ranges from 0 (impossible) to 1 (necessary). Such a probability measure reflects data that has already been collected, and a frequentist approach works provided there is an accurate record of the gender of all students. However, in some cases this may not be possible because the data does not exist, or the accuracy of the data cannot be relied upon. In such cases we have to reason under conditions of uncertainty, where we may need to allocate provisional measures of belief in certain facts before we can draw conclusions. For instance, if an

Intelligent Bioinformatics   Edward Keedwell and Ajit Narayanan
© 2005 John Wiley & Sons, Ltd

insurance company has to decide what the insurance premium should be to cover a pharmaceutical company that is planning to introduce a new anti-cancer drug, with the possibility of toxic side-effects not yet known for the population at large, the insurance company will lose business if it adopts a 'wait-and-see' policy before it sets its premium, especially if national law insists that the pharmaceutical company has to have insurance policies in place before the drug can be released. In such cases the insurance company must try to work out a competitive premium based on what is known as well as what it believes it knows, and hope it gets it right. The insurance company needs a formalism that will allow it to play around with various hypotheses that will allow it to calculate 'best-case' and 'worst-case' scenarios, where such scenarios will make assumptions about mortality rates and toxic side-effects as well as a range of compensation claims that may arise. Conditional probability approaches are widely used to deal with such uncertain situations.

Similarly, there may be uncertainty as to the cause of a particular event. Let us say that the insurance company is presented with a claim from an individual that taking the anti-cancer drug has led to severe side-effects, including loss of energy and therefore loss of job. The company will need to work out the probability that the drug is to blame given the loss of energy and other factors, such as natural ageing or the original cancer having caused bodily damage before the drug was administered for the first time. Frequentist data may be missing when various conditions affect an individual in specific ways.

Related concepts here are those of *independent* and *dependent* events. Two events are independent if the probability of either of them remains the same if the experiment is repeated many times. For instance, the event of 'the coin will land heads' will remain at 50 per cent, no matter how often the coin is flipped, assuming the coin is fair. If the first time the coin is flipped (first event) it lands on heads, there is still a 50–50 chance that the next time it is flipped (second event) it will land on heads, and the next time, and the next time, and so on. While the *sequence* of flipping the coin 20 times and it landing on heads each time may have very low probability, each time the coin is flipped there is a 50–50 chance of it landing on heads. The result of a specific coin flip event is *independent* of the result of the previous coin-flip event. Compare this with 20 coins in a bag, 10 American coins and 10 British coins. The event of taking a coin out of the bag, with the result being an American coin, is 50–50; but if the coin is not put back in the bag the chance of the same event ('the event of the coin being American') is reduced the next time the experiment is repeated, since there are fewer American coins in comparison to British coins. The outcome of the second event is *dependent* on the outcome of the first.

There is therefore a difference between *joint probability* and *conditional probability* when dealing with sequences of events. In the case of a coin being flipped, the joint probability of a sequence of four consecutive flips resulting in four heads is the product of each flip independently of the other flips, i.e. $1/2 * 1/2 * 1/2 * 1/2 = 0.0625$. The probability of each event is multiplied by the probability of the next event in the sequence, and so on, until the end of the sequence is reached. If the four flips are represented by A, B, C and D, respectively, the probability of four consecutive heads is written as $P(A, B, C, D)$ which is calculated as $P(A) * P(B) * P(C) * P(D)$. The events here are all independent of each other. However, the sequence of four American coins being extracted from the bag one after another, without replacement of the coins, consists of dependent events whereby the probability of a later event must take into account the probability of an earlier event. That is, if there are 10 American and 10 British coins in a bag, the probability of the first event is $1/2$, but the probability of the second event has to take into account the probability that an American coin was removed in the previous event. The probability of the second coin being American is reduced and is now $\frac{9}{20}$. The probability sequence therefore is $1/2 * \frac{9}{20} * \frac{8}{20} * \frac{7}{20}$, which is 0.0315. If A, B, C and D represent the four events of taking a coin from the bag, this sequence can be represented as $A * B \mid A * C \mid B * D \mid C$, where '$\mid$' stands for 'given' or 'depending on'. That is, the probability of A, B, C and D, written as $P(A, B, C, D)$ is now $P(A) * P(B \mid A) * P(C \mid AB) * P(D \mid ABC)$, where $P(X \mid YZ...)$ means that the probability of X depends on the probability of Y and Z and $...$ occurring in sequence or as a chain of events.

4.2 Bayes' Theorem

Examining what $P(B \mid A)$ is in the above example, while the result is $\frac{9}{20}$, another way to express this is as follows:

$$P(B \mid A) = \frac{P(AB)}{P(A)}$$

where $P(AB)$ is the joint probability of A and B occurring. In other words, for this example above,

$$P(B \mid A) = \frac{P(AB)}{P(A)} = \frac{\frac{1}{2} * \frac{9}{20}}{\frac{1}{2}} = \frac{9}{20}.$$

Some simple algebraic manipulation then follows:

$$P(B \mid A) = \frac{P(AB)}{P(A)}$$
$$\Rightarrow P(AB) = P(A) \times P(B \mid A)$$
$$\Rightarrow P(AB) = P(B) \times P(A \mid B)$$
$$\Rightarrow P(A \mid B) = \frac{P(A) \times P(B \mid A)}{P(B)}$$
$$\Rightarrow P(A \mid B) = \frac{P(B \mid A) \times P(A)}{P(B)}.$$

In other words, the probability of an event B occurring given that A has occurred has been transformed into a probability of an event A occurring given B has occurred. This is Bayes' Theorem. More formally, Bayes' Theorem states:

$$P(H \mid E) = \frac{P(E \mid H) \times P(H)}{P(E)}$$

where $P(H \mid E)$ is the *posterior probability* of a hypothesis H after considering the evidence E, $P(E \mid H)$ is the *likelihood* and gives the probability of the evidence E assuming H (the conditional probability), $P(H)$ is the prior probability of H alone, and $P(E)$ is a normalizing or scaling constant to ensure that the posterior probability adds up to 1.

Bayes' Theorem is very useful when reasoning under conditions of uncertainty, since it allows us to reason about the prior event H if a subsequent event E has occurred but we do not know whether event H has in fact occurred. For instance, given a bag with 10 British and 5 American coins, if only the event E is observed of a second coin being removed from the bag being American, we can still infer the probability of H being an American coin removed as a first event, as follows (where FCA is 'first coin American' and SCA is 'second coin American'):

$$P(H \mid E) = \frac{P(E \mid H) \times P(H)}{P(E)}$$
$$\Rightarrow P(FCA \mid SCA) = \frac{P(SCA \mid FCA) \times P(FCA)}{P(SCA)}.$$

To calculate this probability a *probability tree* is drawn, as in Figure 4.1, which identifies all possible outcomes. It is assumed that coins are not

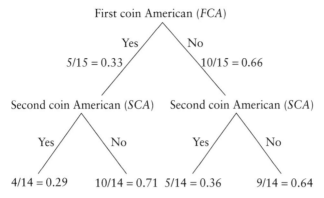

First coin American (*FCA*)

Yes
5/15 = 0.33

No
10/15 = 0.66

Second coin American (*SCA*)   Second coin American (*SCA*)

Yes   No   Yes   No

4/14 = 0.29   10/14 = 0.71   5/14 = 0.36   9/14 = 0.64

Figure 4.1 A probability tree that describes all possible situations when there are 15 coins in a bag of which five are American and 10 are British

replaced in the bag after being extracted. Hence, at the first level of the tree there is a 0.33 probability that the first coin is American and 0.66 probability that the first coin is British. Once the first coin is taken from the bag, the second level of the tree describes the probabilities of the second coin being American, taking into account the two possibilities at the level above. For example, if the first coin had been British (10/15), the chances of the second coin also being British are 9/14. Bayes' Theorem allows reasoning over what the chances of the first coin being American were if only an American coin was observed being taken from the bag at the second stage (as a second event). This is reasoning under uncertainty. The leaves of the tree (bottom-most layer) can be referred to as '*SCA* = yes|*FCA* = yes', '*SCA* = no|*FCA* = yes', '*SCA* = yes|*FCA* = no' and '*SCA* = no|*FCA* = no', reading from left-to-right respectively.

Once this tree is available, the probability of whether the first coin was American can be calculated as follows (all subsequent calculations are rounded to two significant places):

$$P(FCA \mid SCA) = \frac{P(SCA \mid FCA) \times P(FCA)}{P(SCA)}$$

$$\Rightarrow P(FCA \mid SCA) = \frac{0.29 \times 0.33}{P(SCA)}.$$

That is $P(SCA|FCA)$, which is 0.29 (the bottom left-hand 'yes' branch) in Figure 4.1, is multiplied by $P(FCA)$ alone (the top left-hand 'yes' branch). In other words, '$P(X \mid Y)$' means the probability to be found on the branch under node X which in turn is under node Y in the probability tree. To calculate $P(SCA)$ – the denominator – is more complex. There are two possibilities: the bottom left 'yes' branch, and the third from left bottom 'yes' branch. That is, the second coin being American has to take into account both that the first coin was American and that the first coin was not American. In other words, $P(SCA)$ as denominator has to take into account $P(SCA \mid FCA = \text{yes})$ and $P(SCA \mid \text{FCA} = \text{no})$. $P(SCA \mid FCA = \text{yes})$ is the joint probability $P(SCA \mid FCA = \text{yes}) \times P(FCA = \text{yes})$, while $P(SCA \mid FCA = \text{no})$ is the joint probability of $P(SCA \mid FCA = \text{no}) \times P(FCA = \text{no})$. Putting all this into the formula gives:

$$P(FCA \mid SCA) = \frac{0.29 \times 0.33}{P(SCA)}$$

$$\Rightarrow P(FCA \mid SCA) = \frac{0.29 \times 0.33}{P(SCA \mid FCA = \text{yes}) + P(SCA \mid FCA = \text{no})}$$

$$\Rightarrow P(FCA \mid SCA) = \frac{0.29 \times 0.33}{(0.29 \times 0.33) + (0.36 \times 0.66)}$$

$$\Rightarrow P(FCA \mid SCA) = \frac{0.1}{0.1 + 0.22}$$

$$\Rightarrow P(FCA \mid SCA) = \frac{0.1}{0.32} = 0.31.$$

In other words, if the second coin that is taken from the bag is seen to be American, then there is a 31 per cent chance that the first coin was also American (hence a 69 per cent chance that the first coin was British).

Another advantage of Bayes' Theorem is that it can take into account new evidence. Consider the following example. A drugs manufacturer claims that its random roadside drug test will detect the presence of cannabis, cocaine and other drugs in the blood (i.e. show positive for a driver who has taken drugs in the last 72 h) 90 per cent of the time. However, the manufacturer admits that 15 per cent of all drug-free drivers also test positive. A national survey indicates that 20 per cent of all drivers have taken drugs during the last 72 h. One of your friends has just told you that she was recently stopped by the police and the roadside drug test showed positive. She denies having taken drugs. Bayes' Theorem can be used to calculate the probability that your friend took drugs during the 72 h preceding the drugs test. First, draw the probability tree (Figure 4.2, non-italic figures). Then apply Bayes' Theorem, assuming that H is having taken drugs (TD) and E is testing positive (TP). That is, the probability of your friend

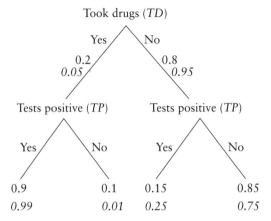

Took drugs (TD)

Figure 4.2 Bayes' Theorem can also take into account new information (new information in italics)

having taken drugs given that the random roadside test showed positive is calculated as follows:

$$P(H \mid E) = \frac{P(E \mid H) \times P(H)}{P(E)}$$

$$\Rightarrow P(TD \mid TP) = \frac{P(TP \mid TD) \times P(TD)}{P(TP)}$$

$$\Rightarrow P(TD \mid TP) = \frac{0.9 \times 0.2}{P(TP)}.$$

To calculate TP, take into account the two possibilities of testing positive having taken drugs and not having taken drugs:

$$P(TD \mid TP) = \frac{0.9 \times 0.2}{P(TP)}$$

$$\Rightarrow P(TD \mid TP) = \frac{0.9 \times 0.2}{P(TP \mid TD = \text{yes}) + P(TP \mid TD = \text{no})}$$

$$\Rightarrow P(TD \mid TP) = \frac{0.9 \times 0.2}{(0.9 \times 0.2) + (0.15 \times 0.8)}$$

$$\Rightarrow P(TD \mid TP) = \frac{0.18}{0.18 + 0.12} = \frac{0.18}{0.3} = 0.6.$$

In other words, there is a 60 per cent chance that your friend did indeed take drugs 72 h prior to the roadside test and only a 40 per cent chance that she is telling the truth. Now imagine that new information arrives that the roadside drug test will now show positive for drivers who have taken drugs 99.9 per cent of the time but that the number of drug-free drivers showing positive has gone up to 25 per cent (Figure 4.2, new probabilities in *italics* under TP at the leaves of the tree). It is a simple matter to enter the new values into the above equations:

$$P(TD \mid TP) = \frac{0.99 \times 0.2}{(0.99 \times 0.2) + (0.25 \times 0.8)}$$

$$= \frac{0.198}{0.198 + 0.2} = \frac{0.198}{0.398} = 0.5$$

That is, the new information increases the chances of your friend telling the truth to 50–50.

If even more recent information arrives that indicates that the original survey of the number of drivers who have taken drugs was wrong (20 per cent) and that the revised figure should be 5 per cent (Figure 4.2, italic figures under TD), this can also be incorporated:

$$P(TD \mid TP) = \frac{0.99 \times 0.05}{(0.99 \times 0.05) + (0.25 \times 0.95)}$$

$$= \frac{0.05}{0.05 + 0.24} = \frac{0.05}{0.29} = 0.17$$

That is, the new information now increases the probability that your friend is telling the truth to 83 per cent. This dramatic improvement in the probability that she is telling the truth results from the high false positive rate as well as reduced chances that she drove after taking drugs.

Finally, Bayes' Theorem can also be used to calculate what sort of false positive rate is required to ensure that drivers who test positive after a random roadside drug test are at least 80 per cent certain to have taken drugs, taking all the new information into account. Try a false positive rate of 6 per cent:

$$P(TD \mid TP) = \frac{0.99 \times 0.05}{(0.99 \times 0.05) + (0.06 \times 0.95)}$$

$$= \frac{0.05}{0.05 + 0.06} = \frac{0.05}{0.11} = 0.45$$

The false positive rate is not low enough, so try 2 per cent:

$$P(TD \mid TP) = \frac{0.99 \times 0.05}{(0.99 \times 0.05) + (0.02 \times 0.95)}$$

$$= \frac{0.05}{0.05 + 0.02} = \frac{0.05}{0.07} = 0.71$$

In fact, a false positive rate of 1 per cent is required to reach the figure of being at least 80 per cent certain that drivers who are randomly tested have indeed taken drugs:

$$P(TD \mid TP) = \frac{0.99 \times 0.05}{(0.99 \times 0.05) + (0.01 \times 0.95)}$$
$$= \frac{0.05}{0.05 + 0.01} = \frac{0.05}{0.06} = 0.83$$

The requirement for such a low false positive rate is a consequence of only 5 per cent of drivers taking drugs, according to the survey.

4.3 Bayesian networks

Bayes' Theorem can also be generalized to deal with belief *networks* (e.g. Delcher *et al.*, 1993). Formally, a Bayesian network is a directed (each arc is an arrow), acyclic (no loops are possible) graph where nodes represent features or attributes (called random variables), arcs denote dependencies as given by some set of rules and the root node is the start node with no incoming links. Also required is a prior probability table for each variable and conditional probabilities to link together all attributes. That is, a node X is linked to another node Y provided there is direct influence of X on Y (in which case the arrow is from X to Y).

For instance, if an insurance company has to decide how to calculate an insurance premium to cover a pharmaceutical company that is planning to introduce a new anti-cancer drug, with the possibility of toxic side-effects not yet known for the population at large, the insurance company can provide a basic set of rules, with hypothetical probabilities. So, for example, the following rules may describe one scenario. 'If the insurance company sets the premium at $50 million dollars a year the drug will be released. If the anti-cancer drug is released, it may cure the cancer. If the drug is released and given to a patient, the patient may die. If a patient dies after receiving the drug, there may be a claim made against the drug company by the patient's relatives. If a claim is made against the drug company, the insurance company may have to pay out more than a million dollars'. This belief network is represented in Figure 4.3. The nodes and links represent rule-based relationships between attributes, and conditional probabilities are assigned to link pairs of nodes together in the network. Once the network is configured, the probabilities of a hypothesis, such as 'premium set at $50m', or whether a patient has died, can

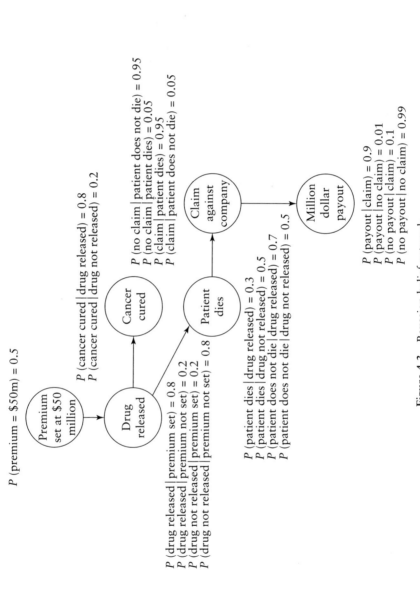

P (premium = $50m) = 0.5

P (cancer cured | drug released) = 0.8
P (cancer cured | drug not released) = 0.2

P (no claim | patient does not die) = 0.95
P (no claim | patient dies) = 0.05
P (claim | patient dies) = 0.95
P (claim | patient does not die) = 0.05

P (drug released | premium set) = 0.8
P (drug released | premium not set) = 0.2
P (drug not released | premium set) = 0.2
P (drug not released | premium not set) = 0.8

P (patient dies | drug released) = 0.3
P (patient dies | drug not released) = 0.5
P (patient does not die | drug released) = 0.7
P (patient does not die | drug not released) = 0.5

P (payout | claim) = 0.9
P (payout | no claim) = 0.01
P (no payout | claim) = 0.1
P (no payout | no claim) = 0.99

Premium set at $50 million

Cancer cured

Drug released

Claim against company

Patient dies

Million dollar payout

Figure 4.3 Bayesian belief network

be calculated from an event such as a million dollar payout having been made. Probabilities and conditional probabilities can then be attached to this belief network.

Now imagine the event 'payout of more than a million dollars made'. What are the implications for P(premium = \$50m)? Now start working backwards. First examine 'claim against company', i.e.

P(payout | claim) = 0.9 and P(payout | no claim) = 0.01.

Continue to work backwards through the network, i.e.

P(claim | patient dies) = 0.95,

P(claim | patient does not die) = 0.05,

P(no claim | patient dies) = 0.05, and

P(no claim | patient does not die) = 0.95.

For patients, continue identifying the conditional probabilities:

P(patient dies | drug released) = 0.3,

P(patient dies | drug not released) = 0.5,

P(patient does not die | drug released) = 0.7, and

P(patient does not die | drug not released) = 0.5.

Similarly, follow the chain backwards through drug released and drug not released until 'premium set' is reached. Combine these probabilities:

P(million dollar payout, claim against company, patient dies, drug released, premium set at \$50m) =

P(million dollar payout) $\times$ P(million dollar payout | claim against company) $\times$ P(claim against company | patient dies) $\times$ P(patient dies | drug released) $\times$ P(drug released | premium set at \$50m).

One particular path through the network is:

'million dollar payout' = 0.9,

'claim against company | patient dies' = 0.95,

'patient dies | drug released' = 0.3,

'drug released | premium set' = 0.8, and

'premium set at $500m' = 0.5,

which when multiplied together gives $0.9 \times 0.95 \times 0.3 \times 0.8 \times 0.5 = 0.103$. This combined probability is added to all other probabilities resulting from all other paths for 'premium set at $50m' to give an overall probability for 'premium set at $50m'. At that stage the insurance company can decide whether it has confidence in its original hypothesis that the premium should be set at $50m, taking into account the probabilities of all conditional probabilities in the network. That is, if the resulting probabilities from all paths sum to a probability greater than 0.5 for 'premium set at $50m', the insurance company has some assurance that it has calculated the probabilities appropriately. For instance, assuming that the interest is only in the implications of a payout having been made for whether a patient has died, four paths are generated:

(payout | claim = 0.9) × (claim | patient dies = 0.95) = 0.885

(payout | no claim = 0.01) × (no claim | patient dies = 0.05) = 0

(payout | claim = 0.9) × (claim | patient does not die = 0.05) = 0.045

(payout | no claim = 0.01) × (no claim | patient does not die = 0.95) = 0.01

To determine the probability of the patient having died, add together those probabilities that have the same hypothesis, i.e.

'patient dies' = 0.885 + 0 = 0.885, and

'patient does not die' = 0.045 + 0.01 = 0.055.

That is, if a payout has been made, it is more likely that the patient has died (0.885) than that the patient has not died (0.055). In this case, the probabilities do not add to 1, and Bayesian networks usually adopt some additional normalization procedure to ensure that the different states of a hypothesis always sum to 1. What has been described here is known as a 'naïve' Bayesian approach, since it assumes that all the variables that appear in the network are totally independent of each other (that there are no statistical dependencies, apart from the conditional probabilities, between any of the variables of features). This is unlikely to be the case in real-world situations.

The main problem with Bayesian belief networks, as seen in the above example, is that the number of paths can grow exponentially. There are 128 paths to be checked (two for 'payout', four for 'claim' and 'no claim', four for 'patient dies' and 'patient does not die', and four for 'drug released' and 'drug not released'), assuming that the only interest is in checking whether the hypothesis 'premium set at $50m dollars' is correct. However, if 'premium set' has a number of different values that need individual checking, the number of paths will grow. Therefore some heuristic methods for searching graphs must be adopted to ensure that Bayesian networks remain tractable when networks have a large number of nodes.

Also, the issue of where the initial assignment of conditional probabilities to the network comes from has not been mentioned. These may have to be extracted from the insurance company's archived data of previously made claims for other products, and therefore there will always be uncertainty as to whether the probabilities assigned for a new product are appropriate.

Application of Bayes' Theorem in artificial intelligence and bioinformatics

As seen from this example, Bayes' Theorem allows reasoning on possible causes after receiving the data. Another way to put this is to say that Bayes' Theorem, with a slight reinterpretation, allows reasoning of the form:

$$P(\text{cause}|\text{effect}) = [P(\text{effect}|\text{cause}) \times P(\text{cause})]/P(\text{effect}).$$

Some of the earliest applications of Bayes' Theorem in artificial intelligence were in fact in the medical domain where knowledge of conditional probabilities concerning causal relationships in medicine were used to derive probabilities of diagnosis (e.g. Pathfinder (Heckerman and Nathwani, 1992); see http://www-users.cs.york.ac.uk/~sara/reference/bayesnets/Software/bnprojects.html for more details of other projects). Bayes' Theorem has found several other applications in artificial intelligence and a good source of material on Bayes' Theorem and such applications, including in the medical domain, can be found at http://www.aaai.org/AITopics/html/uncert.html. Applications in bioinformatics are

more scarce, but a good reference source is http://zlab.bu.edu/kasif/
bayes-net.html, where several links to work on Bayesian networks in
computational molecular biology and bioinformatics can be found, including references to recent papers on Bayesian approaches to gene expression analysis and biological data integration. Most of this work has
appeared in the last four or five years, suggesting a reawakening of interest among bioinformaticians in the application of Bayesian reasoning
to a number of problem areas.

4.4 Markov networks

The Bayesian examples introduced in the previous section dealt with
situations where it was important to identify the probability of hypotheses given evidence. While Bayesian networks can be adapted to deal
with probabilistic *sequences*, another formalism needs to be found if
such sequences are to be modelled with networks that have loops, given
the exponential aspect of calculating Bayesian conditional probabilities.
Markov networks are generally considered more appropriate for dealing with sequences and loops. For example, consider the probabilistic
Markov network in Figure 4.4 and associated *probabilistic transition
matrix* in Table 4.1.

In addition to the normal probabilistic state transitions probabilities can also be attached to the start state of the network (in square

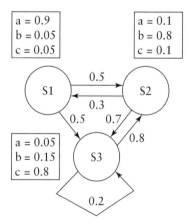

Figure 4.4   A simple probabilistic network, with the transition probabilities specified in the probabilistic transition matrix in Table 4.1 (the probabilities within rectangles represent the probabilities of producing symbols
within each state)

Table 4.1   A probabilistic transition matrix for the Markov graph in Figure 4.4. The rows specify the probability of moving from one state to another, including loops (note that the transition probabilities for each row sum to 1; additionally, the *start* probability of each state (given in square parentheses) can be specified to initialize the Markov process)

	S1	S2	S3
S1 [0.9]	0	0.5	0.5
S2 [0.05]	0.3	0.0	0.7
S3 [0.05]	0	0.8	0.2

parentheses in Table 4.1). A sequence of states, such as S1, S2, S1, S3, S3, S2, S1 can now be given a probability, as follows: $P(S1, S2, S1, S3, S3, S2, S1) = P(S1 \times S2 \mid S1 \times S1 \mid S2 \times S3 \mid S2 \times S3 \mid S3 \times S2 \mid S3 \times S1 \mid S2) = 0.9 \times 0.5 \times 0.3 \times 0.5 \times 0.2 \times 0.8 \times 0.3 = 0.00324$. That is, given that the start of the sequence has probability 0.9, the probability of this particular sequence of states is the product of the transition probabilities of moving from state to state, as given in Table 4.1.

If one symbol is attached to each state (that is, the Markov model produces one specified symbol every time it enters a state), such as 'a' for S1, 'b' for S2 and 'c' for S3, then the sequence S1, S2, S1, S3, S3, S2, S1 produces the symbol sequence 'a b a c c b a', again with probability 0.00324, using just the transition probabilities in Table 4.1. When only one symbol is used instead of a state, the probabilities attached to these symbols, and hence the probabilities attached to the transitions between states, can reflect previous occurrences of these symbols next to each other or the desirability of producing symbols probabilistically.

For instance, the transition probability 'S2 | S1', when translated into a symbolic representation such as 'b|a', reflects the probability 0.5 of 'b' following 'a', as observed by examining actual sequences, or as desired output. In other words, the probabilities attached to moving from S1 to S2 and S1 to S3 (0.5 and 0.5, respectively) reflect the probability of 'a' being followed by 'b' (probability 0.5) and by 'c' (0.5), respectively. However, this restricts states to produce only one symbol. More flexibility and power can be added to a Markov model if more than one symbol is associated with a state. That is, each state may itself have a table of symbols that are probabilistically produced in that state.

For instance, in Figure 4.4 each state is augmented by a table that describes the probabilities of producing one of three symbols in that state. So, the sequence 'a b a c c b a' (state sequence S1, S2, S1, S3, S3,

S2, S1), which has probability of 0.00324 if only one symbol is produced in each state, has actual probability $0.9 \times \mathbf{0.9} \times 0.5 \times \mathbf{0.8} \times 0.3 \times \mathbf{0.9} \times 0.5 \times \mathbf{0.8} \times 0.2 \times \mathbf{0.8} \times 0.8 \times \mathbf{0.8} \times 0.3 \times \mathbf{0.9} = 0.00009675$, where figures in bold give the probability of a particular symbol being produced in a specific state.

In many cases the interest is only in the symbol sequence and the probability of that symbol sequence being generated, without there being a need to know the states passed through. When the states are 'hidden', in that the symbol sequence and its probability are all that is required, a simple form of a 'hidden Markov model' (HMM) results. More formally, an HMM is described as $M = (\alpha, \beta, \pi)$, where α is a table of *transition probabilities* between nodes (for example, the entries in Table 4.1), β is a table of *observation* or *production probabilities* concerning the occurrence of symbols (as given in the tables next to each node in Figure 4.4), and π is a set of initial probabilities (as given in square parentheses in Table 4.1). Just as with automata, an HMM is described as a 'production model' or an 'acceptance model'. A production model will generate a sequence of symbols with a probability as determined by the probability of producing a symbol in a specific state and the probability of moving from one state to another. The overall probability of a sequence is the product of all symbol production/observation probabilities and state transitions.

Such models, in addition to being used for determining the probability of a sequence being accepted or produced, can also be used for *learning*. That is, given a number of sequences for which there is no HMM, the task is to determine an HMM with an appropriate number of states, transition probabilities and symbol occurrence probabilities that best fits all the sequences. A typical problem in bioinformatics may consist of trying to identify the HMM that best fits the four short DNA sequences: AGTC, CAGC, TGC and AGC (note that the sequences need not be the same length). A more powerful Markov model than the simple one described above is required to handle this problem.

HMMs were originally developed in the speech processing domain but were adapted for use in sequence analysis by computer scientists and computational biologists (e.g. Karplus *et al.*, 1997; Eddy, 1998). An HMM in biosequence analysis is *trained* on a set of sequences so that it identifies a *prototype* sequence structure that captures the common elements of the set of sequences. Because looping is allowed, an HMM can be described as a finite model that provides a probability distribution over an infinite number of possible sequences. In bioinformatics, an HMM consists of three *primitives*: match states, insert states and delete states. The match states form the common, prototypical structure, while the insert and delete states permit variations from the prototypical structure. The

Table 4.2   An initial alignment of the four sequences AGTC, CAGC, TGC and AGC, with gaps inserted to form a consensus consisting of AGC (columns 2, 3 and 5), for the construction of a simple HMM

-	A	G	T	C
C	A	G	-	C
T	-	G	-	C
-	A	G	-	C

three primitives can only be connected to each other in three ways. A match state M_i is connected to insert state I_i, delete state D_{i+1} and match state M_{i+1}. An insert state I_i is connected to itself, delete state D_{i+1} and match state M_{i+1}. A delete state D_i is always connected to insert state I_i, delete state D_{i+1} and match state M_{i+1}.[1] A simple HMM for the four sequences above can now be constructed.

First, assume that the four sequences have been initially aligned (Table 4.2). The alignment results in a consensus sequence 'AGC' (columns 2, 3 and 5). One heuristic in building an HMM from scratch is to start with as many match states as there are symbols in the consensus sequence, which in this case is three. Another heuristic is to calculate the average length of the training sequences and to start with as many match states. In the example here, the length of the consensus sequence is used and therefore three match states are chosen. Once the consensus sequence AGC has been found, the empty HMM can be constructed consisting of three match (M) states (one for each symbol of the consensus), four insert (I) states and three delete (D) states (Figure 4.5(a)), following the rules for structuring HMMs. The consensus symbols can then be inserted into each match state. The first sequence AGTC is then entered (Figure 4.5(b)). The path followed by AGTC is given by thick arrows, with the symbols inserted into the appropriate states. After 'begin', A is matched against M1, G is matched against M2, and T, since it cannot be matched against M3, requires a transition to I2, followed by a match of C against M3. The second sequence CAGC is then entered (Figure 4.5(c)). Since the first symbol C cannot be matched against M1, a transition to I0 is required, followed by three matches of A, G and C against M1, M2 and M3, respectively. A note is kept of the transitions

---

[1] This definition of HMMs is taken from the topology used in SAM, the Sequence Alignment and Modelling program suite for the construction of HMMs developed at UCSC (Hughey and Krogh, 1995). It differs slightly from the standard HMM definitions found in the literature by allowing delete, match and insert states to form columns, rather than be staggered, as required by the standard HMM definitions. SAM's definitions are used here because of the intuitive connection of columns in the HMM to columns of a multiple alignment.

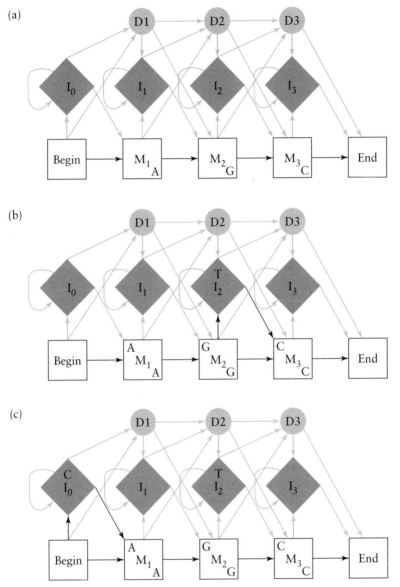

Figure 4.5   The first part of the construction of an HMM for the four sequences
AGTC, CAGC, TGC and AGC

followed to calculate transition probabilities at the end of the process
(Figure 4.7).

The third sequence TGC is entered (Figure 4.6(a)). Since T does not
match M1, a transition to I0 is required to insert T. T now joins C (from
the second sequence) in I0. Since the next symbol is G and a transition to
I1 from I0 is not permitted, a transition to D1 to signify that the consensus

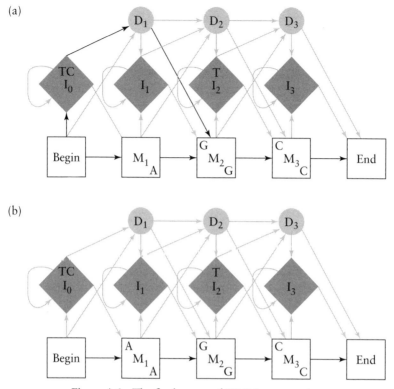

Figure 4.6 The final stages of HMM construction

symbol A has been deleted is made and G is then matched to M2. C is matched to M3. Finally, the fourth sequence AGC matches all three match states Figure 4.6(b). The HMM construction is now complete, with all occurrences of symbols observed. The final and full HMM is given in Figure 4.7. After the final sequence is fed through the HMM, the construction is complete and all probabilities are output together with the HMM (Figure 4.7). At the top left of Figure 4.7 are the four sequences, together with the possible multiple alignment that identifies the consensus AGC. Below each match state M1, M2 and M3 in the HMM are the consensus symbols (with high probability), with token probabilities attached to other symbols not encountered as a consensus. To the left are the insertion probabilities for each insert state. Since I0 is entered twice (for CAGC and TGC), C and T have probabilities close to 0.5 (0.45), with token probabilities attached to the other symbols (X signifies any other symbol). T has a high probability in I2 to signify it was inserted in at least one sequence. At the bottom of the figure are the paths traced by each sequence. Links not used for modelling any sequence are given in dashed lines, while solid lines indicate that a

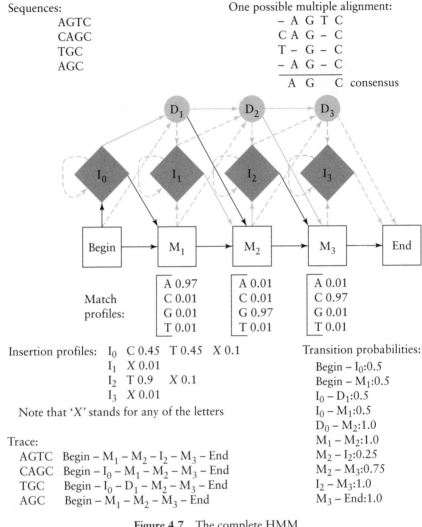

Sequences: One possible multiple alignment:
  AGTC   – A G T C
  CAGC   C A G – C
  TGC   T – G – C
  AGC   – A G – C
                                                A G   C   consensus

Match
profiles:

A 0.97	A 0.01	A 0.01
C 0.01	C 0.01	C 0.97
G 0.01	G 0.97	G 0.01
T 0.01	T 0.01	T 0.01

Insertion profiles: I_0 C 0.45   T 0.45   X 0.1   Transition probabilities:
                     I_1 X 0.01   Begin – I_0:0.5
                     I_2 T 0.9   X 0.1   Begin – M_1:0.5
                     I_3 X 0.01 I_0 – D_1:0.5
Note that 'X' stands for any of the letters I_0 – M_1:0.5
                                                            D_0 – M_2:1.0
Trace: M_1 – M_2:1.0
  AGTC Begin – M_1 – M_2 – I_2 – M_3 – End M_2 – I_2:0.25
  CAGC Begin – I_0 – M_1 – M_2 – M_3 – End M_2 – M_3:0.75
  TGC   Begin – I_0 – D_1 – M_2 – M_3 – End I_2 – M_3:1.0
  AGC   Begin – M_1 – M_2 – M_3 – End M_3 – End:1.0

Figure 4.7   The complete HMM

particular link was used. To the right below the HMM are the transition probabilities, calculated on the basis of how often that link was followed for the four sequences. For instance, the link between 'begin' and I0 has a 0.5 transition probability because this link was followed for two of the four sequences. Also, the links between I0 and D1 and I0 and M1 have 0.5 transition probability each because, of the two sequences that entered I0, one exited to D1 and the other to M1. Some links have probability 1 to signify that all the sequences that entered that state also exited by that link. The links between M2 and I2 and M2 and M3 have 0.25 and 0.75

probability to reflect that three of the strands exited to M3 and only one to I2. Delete states have 0 probability since they do not emit any symbols. This HMM is then said to 'model' the four sequences, and the probabilities of each sequence can now be determined as the product of all the probabilities along its path. For instance, for AGTC:

$$AGTC = 0.5 \times 0.97 \times 1.0 \times 0.97 \times 0.25 \times 0.9 \times 1.0 \times 0.97 \times 1.0$$
$$= 0.102676$$

That is, from left to right, 0.5 represents the link between 'begin' and M1, 0.97 the probability of matching A in M1, 1.0 the link between M1 and M2, 0.97 the match between G and M2, 0.25 is the link between M2 and I2, 0.9 the probability of inserting T in I2, 1.0 the link between I2 and M3, 0.97 the match between C and M3, and finally 1.0 the link between M3 and 'end'.

One of the benefits of an HMM is that the model can be used to generate other sequences not so far explicitly represented. For instance, following only the links that have been activated when evaluating the four previous sequences, the 'new' sequence CAGTC is also a sequence of the model if the two insert states are both entered for a sequence:

$$CAGTC = 0.5 \times 0.45 \times 0.5 \times 0.97 \times 1.0 \times 0.97 \times 0.25 \times 0.9$$
$$\times 1.0 \times 0.97 \times 1.0 = 0.023103.$$

One of the problems with HMMs and any probabilistic approach that uses products of probabilities is that resulting probabilities become increasingly smaller with each link or state probability. For an HMM consisting of 40 or 50 match states and associated insert and delete states with links (that is, for an HMM that deals with sequences that are on average 40 or 50 symbols long or whose consensus is between 40 and 50 symbols), the probabilities of sequences may become so small as to become almost meaningless. Also, some computers may not be able to calculate extremely small numbers with accuracy. For this reason *log-odds scoring* is often used, whereby each sequence is considered as a random collection of symbols, the null model. The null model can then be used to assign a DNA sequence of length L a probability of 0.25^L, where each nucleotide has a 0.25 random chance of appearing (or 0.05^L if dealing with amino acid sequences). The log-odds score for a sequence S can then be calculated as:

$$\log \frac{P(S)}{0.25^L} = \log P(S) - L \log 0.25$$

For instance, the logs-odd score for CAGTC is:

$$\log \frac{P(CAGTC)}{0.25^L} = \log P(CAGTC) - L \log 0.25$$
$$= \log 0.023103 - (5 \times \log 0.25)$$
$$= -3.7677928 - (5 \times -1.3862944)$$
$$= -3.7677928 + 6.93147181$$
$$= 3.16367901 \text{ (using natural logs)}$$

That is, the HMM probability of CAGTC is 0.023103, and from this is subtracted (with logs, dividing x by y becomes subtracting y from x) five (the length of the sequence) times the random chance of the sequence being random (with logs, raising to the power becomes multiplication). The final result can be rounded to 3.164. The above calculation was undertaken after the probability of CAGTC was calculated, but the log-odds formula can be applied from the beginning of a sequence as it enters the HMM so that a running natural log score can be maintained as the symbols are processed one by one and insert, match and transition probabilities are applied.

Three major advantages with HMMs are that conserved regions of sequences (subsequences that occur in all strings, such as the same gene across a number of different organisms, that can therefore be assumed to be conserved through evolution) are modelled very well, that deletion and insertion of nucleotides and amino acids are explicitly represented in the HMM and that the actual states passed through by the HMM are hidden from the user who may only be interested in the final probabilities. This example assumed that sequences were already aligned before presentation to the HMM. In fact, HMMs can also be used to construct alignments, and methods such as the Viterbi algorithm (with variations) exist for this purpose.

Applications of HMMs in bioinformatics

HMMs can be considered a true bioinformatics technique, with several applications in profile family characterization in homology search, gene finding (see Colin Cherry's *HMMs in Bioinformatics*, http://www. cs.ualberta.ca/~colinc/cmput606/606FinalPres.ppt). One of the best sources for further information is the ISMB99 Tutorial on HMMs by Melissa Kline, Christian Barrett and Kevin Karplus (http://www.

cse.ucsc.edu/research/compbio/ismb99.tutorial.html). This page also contains links to other HMM-related pages.

4.5 Summary of chapter

1 Probability is playing an increasingly important role in artificial intelligence and the ability of systems to reason under conditions of uncertainty. Of particular importance and interest are Bayesian and Hidden Markov Model approaches, which have the ability to calculate the probability of future events and sequences on the basis of past events and sequences. Both approaches use special types of graph for representing information about the domain.

2 At the heart of the Bayesian approach is the concept of 'conditional probability', i.e. the probability of a prior event A having occurred given that a subsequent event B has occurred. If there is a hypothetical causal relationship between A and B, and B is seen to occur but not A, Bayes' Theorem can be used to calculate the probability of A having occurred.

3 The specific hypothetical relationship between A and B above can be generalized to any causal sequences A, B, C, etc. In this case we may have multiple possible causes of particular events and long sequences of causal events. Bayesian networks are special types of graph that allow the calculation of prior events in a multiple causal system, but problems exist concerning the tractability of such networks if the graph becomes complex. Nevertheless, Bayesian approaches are suitable for AI and Bioinformatics applications where it is important to reason about the probability of events.

4 Hidden Markov Models (HMMs) can be described formally as a discrete dynamical system governed by a Markov chain that emits a sequence of observable outputs. They are useful for dealing with sequences. A typical HMM consists of three 'layers' of nodes with specific interconnectivity. Typically, the first layer consists of 'match' states that reflect the frequency of commonly occurring symbols in a set of observed sequences, another layer reflects the frequency of new symbols being inserted in specific positions in some of the observed sequences, and the third layer represents the frequency of symbols being deleted from some of the observed sequences.

5   HMMs are particulary useful for dealing with multiple alignments, profiles and various probabilistic models of biological sequences. A number of algorithms now exist for constructing HMMs for optimal multiple alignment. There are typically two phases to constructing an HMM. In the first phase the task is to find a set of transition and emission probabilities that reflect the probability of observing the training sequences. In the second phase the task is to determine the probability that a new sequence belongs to the domain being modelled by the HMM.

4.6 References

Delcher, A., Kasif, S. Goldberg, H. *et al.* (1993) Protein secondary-structure modeling with probabilistic networks. *International Conference on Intelligent Systems and Molecular Biology*, pp. 109–117.

Eddy, S.R. (1998) Profile hidden Markov models. *Bioinformatics* **14** (9), 755–763.

Heckerman, D.E. and Nathwani, B.N, (1992) An evaluation of the diagnostic accuracy of Pathfinder. *Comput. Biomed. Res.*, **25** (1), 56–74.

Hughey, R. and Krogh, A. (1995) SAM: Sequence alignment and modelling software system. Technical Report UCSC-CRL-95-7, University of California, Santa Cruz, CA, January 1995 (regularly updated).

Karplus, K., Sjolander, K., Barrett, C. *et al.* (1997) Predicting protein structure using hidden Markov models. *Proteins, Supplement 1*, 134–139.

Software availability

A good starting point for downloading software for Bayesian reasoning is http://www.ai.mit.edu/~murphyk/Bayes/bnsoft.html, where a number of graphical packages for Bayesian networks are described and compared. The standard HMM software used by bioinformaticians is HMMER (pronounced 'hammer'), from http://hmmer.wustl.edu/. It is written mainly for Unix and Linux platforms, although a Windows version does exist if changes are made to the code.

5
Nearest Neighbour and Clustering Approaches

5.1 Introduction

Consider eight prostate cancer patients who have had biopsies in a clinic, with measurement of two specific genes through gene expression analysis: hepatoma mRNA for the serine protease hepsin (accession number X07732) and the c-myc oncogene (V00568). Doctors at the clinic believe they have a novel way of identifying more accurate therapeutic strategies for individual patients based on these gene expression measurements. Each of the patients then undergoes an individualized therapy regime consisting of varying combinations of androgen suppression and radiation. These therapeutic strategies prove successful, thereby vindicating therapeutic diagnosis on the basis of the measurement of these two genes. A new patient enters the clinic and also has a biopsy. The question now arises as to whether, from previous records of successful therapy, the doctors can predict the sort of therapy that stands most chance of being successful for the new patient, given his gene expression measurements for X07732 and V00568.[1]

A nearest-neighbour approach to this diagnosis problem would be as follows. The quantitative measurements for these two genes are converted to $\log_2$ ratios, ranging from 0 to 6. Each of the eight previous patients is plotted on a two-dimensional graph so that their measurements on these two genes act as x and y coordinates to project each

[1] This example is an adaptation of an example provided by Winston (1992).

Intelligent Bioinformatics   Edward Keedwell and Ajit Narayanan
© 2005 John Wiley & Sons, Ltd

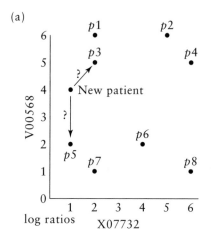

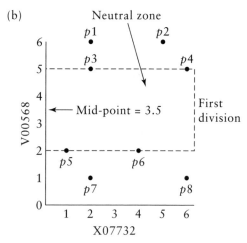

Figure 5.1   The method for constructing a decision tree.

patient's profile onto a two-dimensional space (Figure 5.1(a)). For instance, patient 1 *(p1)* has value 6 on V00568 and value 2 on X07732. The question of how doctors treat the new patient now becomes the question of locating the new patient as close as possible to his neighbour in this two-dimensional space, given the new patient's measurements on the two genes. In other words, the doctors ask who the nearest neighbour of the new patient is. If the doctors can determine who the nearest neighbour is, then they can administer the same therapeutic regime to the new patient as the new patient's nearest neighbour, with the expectation that the therapy stands a better chance of being successful according to previous experience than if they were to come up with a therapeutic regime from scratch.

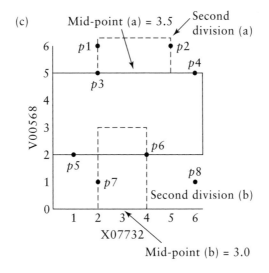

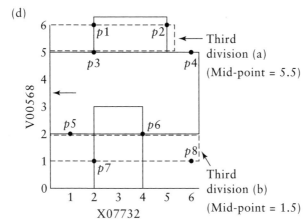

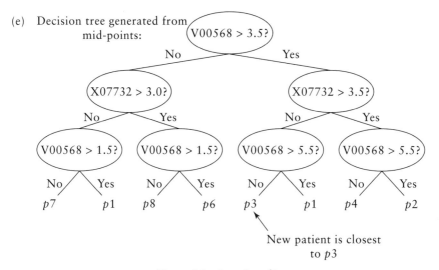

Figure 5.1 (continued)

5.2 Nearest neighbour method

The basis for all nearest neighbour methods is the *consistency heuristic* (Friedman, Bentley and Raphael, 1977; Dasarathy, 1991): (a) find the most similar case, as measured by known properties, for the new case with unknown property (in this case unknown therapeutic regime); (b) then guess that the unknown property of the new case is the same as the property of the most similar case. Nearest neighbour calculations can be performed at run-time, but there are advantages in storing the information on how to determine a nearest neighbour ahead of new samples so that, as new cases enter the system, they can immediately be located nearest to their most similar neighbour. It may seem trivial to undertake a nearest neighbour calculation for this simple example. After all, a simple visual inspection seems to indicate that the new patient's nearest neighbour is *p3* or possibly *p5*. However, imagine that not two genes are measured but 50. There will be a 50-dimensional space that needs examining and visual inspection will no longer be sufficient. The nearest neighbour method provides a systematic method for locating new cases as close as possible to existing cases, irrespective of the number of dimensions, thereby adding some consistency to the decision-making process.

The nearest neighbour method can be described generally as follows. For the cases with known therapeutic strategies, generate a decision tree (Figure 5.1) where each node is connected to a set of possible answers and each non-leaf node is connected to a test which splits its set of possible answers into subsets corresponding to different test results. Each branch will then carry a particular test result's subset to another node. Informally, the idea is to divide up the cases in advance of nearest neighbour calculation so that each patient falls within their own unique space. The two attributes X07732 and V00568 (measurements known for all eight patients plus the new patient) are used repeatedly until only one patient is in each set. The cases are divided in such a way that an equal number of cases falls on either side. The eight cases are first projected onto a two-dimensional space using the attributes (Figure 5.1(a)). The steps are as follows.

1 Use V00568 first and find a point on that dimension that separates the eight cases with a known property (therapeutic strategy) into two equal subsets of four (Figure 5.1(b)). Note that *p3* and *p4* have value 5 on V00568, whereas *p5* and *p6* have value 2 on this dimension. The space between these four patients is the separation between the

top half of the group and the bottom half of the group (four patients in each subgroup). If the average between 2 and 5 is taken the result, 3.5, can be used to determine the *mid-point* that separates the eight cases into two equal subsets of four. The space between is called the *neutral zone*. This is the first division.

2   Next, apply the second dimension, X07732, to each subset (Figure 5.1(c)).

   (a) First ask, for the top group of four patients, what the X07732 mid-point value is that separates that group into two equal subsets of two cases each. For the top group, *p1, p2, p3* and *p4*, the X07732 mid-point value that separates *p1* and *p3* from *p2* and *p4* is 3.5, since *p1* and *p3* have X07732 value two and *p2* (the closer case among *p2* and *p4)* has value five. This is the first division for X07732.

   (b) Also, determine the mid-point value for the lower group. The two cases that are closest to each other are *p7* and *p6* in this group of four and constitute the second and third items, in increasing X07732 value. The mid-point between them is 3. That is where the second division for X07732 takes place.

3   There are now four groups of two cases each. Go back to V00568 to identify a final set of divisions that will uniquely locate each sample into one of eight regions of space (Figure 5.1(d)).

   (a) For the top left group of two *(p1, p3)*, the mid-point is 5.5 (average between 5 and 6). Each case now falls in its own distinct region and no further division is required.

   (b) For the top right group *(p2, p4)*, the mid-point is also 5.5. Each case now falls in its own distinct region and no further division is required.

   (c) For the bottom left group *(p5, p7)*, the mid-point is 1.5, and no further division is required.

   (d) For the bottom right group *(p6, p8)*, the mid-point is also 1.5, and no further division is required.

The first phase of the nearest neighbour method is complete. The second and final stage is to generate a decision tree that reflects the order in which the attributes were applied and the mid-points found (Figure 5.1(e)). The first mid-point is used to root the tree. A 'yes' branch and 'no' branch lead to the second set of tests at the level below. Since there are two mid-points here, they both form separate tests at that level. Finally, place all four mid-point tests at the level below so that, by following the tree and applying the tests, each of the eight cases uniquely falls in a leaf node by itself. To determine the nearest neighbour of the new case, simply apply the root test and follow the appropriate branches to subsequent tests, and so on, until a leaf node is reached, where the most similar case will be found. In this example the nearest neighbour method predicts that the best therapeutic strategy for the new patient is the same as that followed by *p3*.

Typically, nearest neighbour methods do not return just one candidate nearest neighbour but k nearest neighbours, where k is determined by the user. Each of the k nearest neighbours can vote on their confidence as to whether it is the nearest neighbour by calculating some distance metric between itself and the new case. The regions of space around each sample (the neutral zones) can be used for this purpose, since it is possible that a new case falls just one side of a mid-point but is closer in distance to a sample in a bordering region than it is to the sample in the region of space in which it falls.

In general, a decision tree with branching factor two and depth d will have 2^d leaves, where d will have to be large enough to ensure $2^d \geq n$ (where n is the number of samples or objects). Nearest neighbour approaches are particularly useful for dealing with attributes that are known to be 'noisy' or which have values that are often missing, since the decision tree can project a more accurate value for such attributes on the basis of comparing values on attributes that are known to be secure for all samples. Also, the information as to why a new sample is categorized with a nearest neighbour is readily available in the form of a decision tree.

5.3 Nearest neighbour approach for secondary structure protein folding prediction

SIMPA (Levin, Robson and Garner, 1986; Levin, 1997) is an extended nearest neighbour method for predicting the secondary structures of proteins. Consider three short amino acid sequences and their known secondary structure conformations:

h h s s s s c   h s c c c c c   h h s s c c c
A T S L V F W   S T S G V V W   S C N G A F W

For example, the amino acid sequence ATSLVFW has secondary structure hhsssc, where 'h' stands for 'helix', 's' for sheet, and 'c' for coil. (SIMPA uses several other secondary structure conformations.) That is, A and T partake in a helix, S, L, V and F in a sheet and W in a coil. Now imagine that a new, homologous amino acid sequence is encountered (homologous as given by some alignment algorithm) with unknown secondary structure: STNGIYW. The question arises as to whether the secondary structure of this new sequence can be predicted based on a knowledge of the structure of its three homologues.

First, find or construct a similarity matrix, such as that provided in Table 5.1. This table, which describes the similarity and dissimilarity relationships between pairs of amino acids, is used to generate a *conformation matrix* by working through each sequence with known structure and comparing its amino acid constituents with those of the sequence with unknown structure. So, for example, the similarity between STNGIYW (the sequence with unknown secondary structure) and ATSLVFW (the first of

Table 5.1 A hypothetical similarity matrix that identifies the relationships between individual amino acids based on various properties, such as charge, aromaticity and hydrophobicity (adapted from Levin *et al.* (1986)). For example, glycine (G) in the second column of the table is neutral (0) with respect to proline (P, second row) and negatively related to valine (V, thirteenth row) with value −1. Phenylalanine (F) in the third column from the right is positively related to tyrosine (Y, row 19)

	G	P	D	E	A	N	Q	S	T	K	R	H	V	I	M	C	L	F	Y	W
G	2																			
P	0	3																		
D	0	0	2																	
E	0	−1	1	2																
A	0	−1	0	1	2															
N	0	0	1	0	0	3														
Q	0	0	0	1	0	1	2													
S	0	0	0	0	1	0	0	2												
T	0	0	0	0	0	0	0	0	2											
K	0	0	0	0	0	1	0	0	0	2										
R	0	0	0	0	0	0	0	0	0	1	2									
H	0	0	0	0	0	0	0	0	0	0	0	2								
V	−1	−1	−1	−1	0	−1	−1	−1	0	−1	−1	−1	2							
I	−1	−1	−1	−1	0	−1	−1	−1	0	−1	−1	−1	1	2						
M	−1	−1	−1	−1	0	−1	−1	−1	0	−1	−1	−1	0	0	2					
C	0	0	0	0	0	0	0	0	0	0	0	0	0	0	0	2				
L	−1	−1	−1	−1	0	−1	−1	−1	0	−1	−1	−1	1	0	2	0	2			
F	−1	−1	−1	−1	−1	−1	−1	−1	−1	−1	−1	−1	0	1	0	−1	0	2		
Y	−1	−1	−1	−1	−1	−1	−1	−1	−1	−1	−1	0	0	0	0	−1	0	1	2	
W	−1	−1	−1	−1	−1	−1	−1	−1	−1	−1	−1	−1	0	0	0	−1	0	0	0	2

Table 5.2 The conformation prediction table for the three homologues in comparison with the sequence with unknown structure

	h	s	c
Residue 1	$6 + 9 + 9 = 24$		
Residue 2	$6 + 9 = 15$		9
Residue 3		$6 + 9 = 15$	9
Residue 4		$6 + 9 = 15$	9
Residue 5		6	$9 + 9 = 18$
Residue 6		6	$9 + 9 = 18$
Residue 7			$6 + 9 + 9 = 24$

the sequences with known secondary structure) is: $1 + 2 + 0 - 1 + 1 + 1 + 2 = 6$. That is, the similarity between the first symbols of each strand 'S' and 'A' is 1, the second symbols 'T' and 'T' is 2, third symbols 'N' and 'S' is 0, fourth symbols 'G' and 'L' is -1, fifth symbols 'I' and 'V' is 1, sixth symbols 'Y' and 'F' is 1, and final symbols 'W' and 'W' is 2. These pairwise similarity scores are added together to result in a score of 6 for these two sequences. Calculate the scores for STNGIYW and the other two homologues also, giving 9 for STSGVVW $(2 + 2 + 0 + 2 + 1 + 0 + 2)$ and $9(2 + 0 + 2 + 2 + 0 + 1 + 2)$ for SCNGAFW. There are three overall scores that measure the similarity between each of the homologues and the sequence with unknown structure: 6, 9 and 9.

Next, allocate these scores in a *conformation prediction table* for each residue (Table 5.2). The rows of this table describe each residue in the homologue set (residues 1 to 7), and the rows represent the three types of conformation possible (helix, sheet and coil).

For residue 1, all three homologues have the **h** conformation for their first residue, and so each of the overall homologue scores are entered and summed in this column: 6+9+9. For the second residue, the first and the third of the homologues have **h** whereas the second homologue has **c**. The scores for the first and third homologues are inserted under the **h** column (6 and 9, respectively) and the score for the second homologue is inserted under the **c** column (9). For the third residue, the first and third sequences have conformation **s** whereas the second has **c**. The overall scores 6 (for the first homologue) and 9 (for the third homologue) are added under the **s** column whereas the overall score 9 (for the second homologue) is entered under the **c** column. This process is continued for all the residues (Table 5.2). Then, for each residue in the new strand STNGIYW, the conformation with the maximum score is allocated to that residue. For instance, the first symbol in the new strand is 'S'. Looking at the first residue row of Table 5.2, the maximum (and only) score falls under the **h** column. The first residue of the new strand is therefore predicted to partake in a helix conformation. For the second residue, there are two possibilities, with 15 for **h** and 9 for **c**. Since the maximum value is 15, the second residue is predicted to partake in a helix conformation. Applying this maximum function to all the other residues results in a prediction that the new strand STNGIYW has conformation **hhssccc**, i.e. helix, helix, sheet, sheet, coil, coil coil, for its seven amino acid residues.

SIMPA (Levin, 1997) uses a more complex version of this method, adopting a threshold value (minimum score) of 7 before a score can be inserted into the conformation prediction table, a 'moving window' moving one residue along both the new and homologue strands, and additional weightings on the scores in the secondary structure similarity matrix. SIMPA is an extended nearest neighbour technique since it essentially attributes a conformation to a residue in the new sample on the basis of nearest neighbour residues with known conformations in homologues. The conformation here is a *class*, and SIMPA is a procedure that predicts a class c (a conformation in this case) on the basis of the nearest neighbours n (residues in homologues) to a query object q (residues in the new strand).

5.4 Clustering

Nearest neighbour approaches generally work well when there are a few attributes and many samples. The small number of attributes can be used one at a time, in no specific order, to generate a multidimensional space onto which each sample can be projected as a point. If, after one cycle through the small number of attributes, it is not possible to locate each sample in its own unique space, the attributes can be reused over and over until each sample is uniquely located. However, many problems in bioinformatics are characterized by a few samples having very many attributes. For instance, a family of proteins may consists of about 20 actual sequences (samples), each of which can contain very many, possibly hundreds or thousands, of residues (attributes called 'residue 1', 'residue 2', etc.). If the attributes are binary (e.g. 'yes/no', 'on/off') and the number of attributes a is such that $2^a < n$, where n is the number of samples, attributes can be reused (as in Figure 5.1) until a unique sample at each leaf of the decision tree results. However, if there are many more attributes than samples, the problem arises of deciding which attributes to use, since not all of them will need to be used to generate the decision

Table 5.3   A table of four patients with their gene expression measurements across five genes. The gene values are 'absent' and 'present', which are coded in the table as '0' for 'absent' and '1' for present. Patients 1 to 4 are referred to as $p1$–$p4$ in the text

	Gene 1	Gene 2	Gene 3	Gene 4	Gene 5
Patient 1	1	1	0	0	0
Patient 2	1	0	0	0	0
Patient 3	0	0	1	0	0
Patient 4	0	0	1	1	0

tree. This then means that there will be different decision trees depending on which attributes are used. Also, there is the possibility that by arbitrarily choosing some attributes rather than others certain attributes are missed that lead to clear and separate regions of space for each sample. For instance, 'noisy' attributes may be used that do not distinguish the sample well and instead project the samples into a very tight region of space where clear separation is not maintained. For this reason, methods which attempt to take into account the information present in all attributes before projecting each sample into its own region of space are preferred for many bioinformatics problems.

Consider, for instance, four cancer patients $p1$ to $p4$ who are measured across five genes (Table 5.3) that are measured in binary form (e.g. 'gene absent' and 'gene present'). To project each patient into a separate region of space would require only two of the five genes/attributes to be used – but which ones? For instance, if Gene 1 is used, that will separate the four patients into two subgroups of two each ($p1$ and $p2$ on the one hand, and $p3$ and $p4$ on the other), but if Gene 2 is used there will be unequal distribution. Clustering removes the need to make such a decision by using the information present in all five genes in an iterative process.

The first iteration in clustering (Figure 5.2) involves calculating a *matching coefficient* for every pair of patients in the table across all genes/attributes. For instance, the matching coefficient for $p1$ and $p2$ is the number of identical gene expression values they share divided by the total number of genes/attributes. Patient 1 and Patient 2 share identical gene expression values for Gene 1 (this gene is present (1) for both patients), Gene 3 (0), Gene 4 (0) and Gene 5 (0). Therefore, out of five genes, Patient 1 and Patient 2 share four identical values. If score 1 is used for each perfect match and 0 for each mismatch, this produces:

$$p1/p2 = 1 + 0 + 1 + 1 + 1 = 4/5 = 0.8.$$

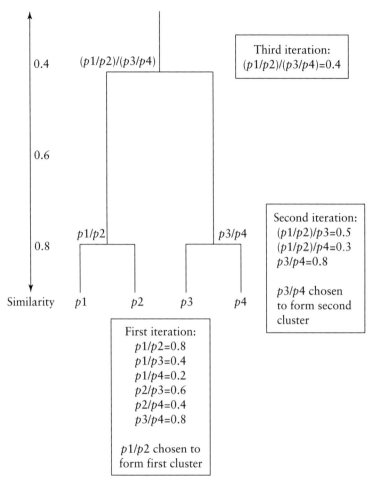

Figure 5.2 A cluster diagram that represents the similarities between four patients *p1–p4* as measured on five genes

where '*p1/p2*' means that *p1* is matched with *p2*. Similarly:

$$p1/p3 = 0 + 0 + 0 + 1 + 1 = 2/5 = 0.4;$$
$$p1/p4 = 0 + 0 + 0 + 0 + 1 = 1/5 = 0.2;$$
$$p2/p3 = 0 + 1 + 0 + 1 + 1 = 3/5 = 0.6;$$
$$p2/p4 = 0 + 1 + 0 + 0 + 1 = 2/5 = 0.4;$$
$$p3/p4 = 1 + 1 + 1 + 0 + 1 = 4/5 = 0.8.$$

There are six pairwise comparisons to be made for four patients in the first iteration. In general, if there are *n* patients or samples, there will be an initial *n − 1 + n − 2 + n − 3 + . . . 2 + 1* comparisons.

The next stage is to choose the match that has the highest matching co-efficient. In this example, there are two values of 0.8 ($p1/p2$ and $p3/p4$). Choose one at random, say $p1/p2$, and form the first *cluster*. The calcula-tion of all pairwise matching coefficients is repeated, but this time using $p1/p2$ as one 'patient' and taking partial matches into account. So, the average matching coefficient for $p1/p2$ and $p3 = 0 + 0.5 + 0 + 1 + 1 = 2.5/5 = 0.5$. That is, there is no match (0 score) for Gene 1, since both $p1$ and $p2$ have value 1 for this gene whereas $p3$ has 0; there is a *par-tial* match between $p1/p2$ and $p3$ for Gene 2, since $p2$ has value 0 and $p3$ has value 0, and this partial match is given a score of 0.5 to indi-cate that one half of $p1/p2$ shares a value with $p3$; there is no match between $p1/p2$ and $p3$ for Gene 3 (0 value); there is a total match be-tween $p1/p2$ and $p3$ for Genes 4 and 5 (score 1 each), giving 2.5 shared values out of five genes, which is 0.5 Similarly, the matching coefficients for $p1/p2$ and $p4 = 0 + 0.5 + 0 + 0 + 1 = 1.5/5 = 0.3$, and for $p3$ and $p4(p3/p4) = 0.8$ (as before). Since $p3/p4$ has the highest coefficient value in the second iteration, they form the second cluster.

The third and final iteration for this example consists of matching the two clusters $p1/p2$ and $p3/p4$ together (that is $p1/p2$ is considered one 'patient', as is $p3/p4$), with partial matches taken into account. The matching coefficient for $(p1/p2)/(p3/p4) = 0 + 0.5 + 0 + 0.5 + 1 = 2/5 = 0.4$. That is, $p1/p2$ has no match whatsoever with $p3/p4$ for Gene 1 (therefore 0 score); for Gene 2 half of $p1/p2$, namely, $p2$, shares a feature (0) with $p3/p4$ (which both share the same feature 0), thereby resulting in 0.5 score; there is no partial match whatsoever on Gene 3 (score 0); half partial match for Gene 4 (0.5 score), and total match on Gene 5 (score 1). This results in an overall matching coefficient of 0.4 for $(p1/p2)/(p3/p4)$.

Since all the individual patients have been combined into one super-cluster, the iterative process is complete. A *similarity tree* is now generated that reflects the order in which the patients were clustered (Figure 5.2) with an indication of the matching coefficient values for each clustering. This form of hierarchical clustering is known as UPGMA (unweighted pair group method with arithmetic mean) (Michener and Sokal, 1957; Sneath and Sokal, 1973).

5.5 Advanced clustering techniques

So far, only samples in Table 5.3 were clustered. However, genes can also be clustered. Imagine an extended version of the data in Table 5.3, but with the difference that each gene now has one of four possible values

Table 5.4 A gene expression sample table, with genes occupying rows and samples columns

	Patient 1	*Patient 2*	*Patient 3*	*Patient 4*
Gene 1	3	2	1	0
Gene 2	2	1	0	1
Gene 3	3	1	0	2
Gene 4	1	0	1	0
Gene 5	0	0	3	3

(0, 1, 2, 3). First, the table is transposed so that genes appear in the rows and samples in the columns (Table 5.4).

The gene profiles can be plotted on a graph, as given in Figure 5.3. That is, each line on the graph connects a gene's values across all patients. The next stage is to identify how similar each gene is to other genes, given the profiles across all samples.

A *Euclidean distance* approach to this calculation is as follows:

$$d(g, g') = \sqrt{\sum_s (e_{gs} - e_{g's})^2}$$

That is, the difference between two genes g and g' is the square root of the summed squares of the differences between an expression value e of g for a sample s and the expression value e of g' for that same sample summed

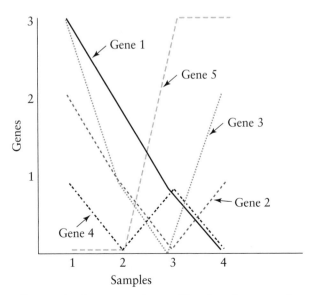

Figure 5.3 Gene expression profiles plotted on a graph

across all samples. The difference is squared to prevent negative values. So, for instance, for the five genes and adopting a pairwise comparison in the first instance:

$$d(g1, g2) = \sqrt{\sum (e_{gs} - e_{g's})^2} = \sqrt{(3-2)^2 + (2-1)^2 + (1-0)^2 + (0-1)^2}$$
$$= \sqrt{1 + 1 + 1 + 1} = 2$$

That is, Gene 1 has values 3, 2, 1 and 0 across the four samples (patients) and Gene 2 has values 2, 1, 0 and 1 for the same four samples. Gene 1 values constitute the first item of each pair of values in the formula, and gene 2 values constitute the second item of each pair. Adopting the Euclidean method, the two genes have a similarity measure of 2 (the closer the similarity measure to 0, the more similar two genes are). The other pairwise comparisons result in:

$d(g1, g2) = 2$ $d(g1, g3) = 2.45$ $d(g1, g4) = 2.83$ $d(g1, g5) = 5.1$
$d(g2, g3) = 1.414$ $d(g2, g4) = 2$ $d(g2, g5) = 4$
$d(g3, g4) = 3.162$ $d(g3, g5) = 4.472$
$d(g4, g5) = 3.742$

A second approach to calculating the differences between pairs of genes is the *Manhattan* approach, defined as follows:

$$d(g, g') = \sum_s |e_{gs} - e_{g's}|$$

That is, the difference between a pair of genes is simply the absolute difference between the expression values across all samples. So, for example,

$$d(g1, g2) = |3 - 2| + |2 - 1| + |1 - 0| + |0 - 1| = 4$$
$$d(g1, g3) = |3 - 3| + |2 - 1| + |1 - 0| + |0 - 2| = 4$$

etc. The Euclidean distance method is adopted here since, as can be seen by comparing g1, g2 and g3 above, the Euclidean distance method can make finer distinctions than the Manhattan method. That is, the Euclidean distance method separates g1 and g2 from g1 and g3 (2 and 2.45, respectively), whereas the Manhattan method gives the same values for each pair (4).

Once the pairwise distance calculations have been made, start merging the genes with closest distance to each other. There are a number of methods for doing this in the literature, but one of the simplest will be used here. Looking at the results of the Euclidean distance calculations for pairs of genes above, there is one pair ($g2$, $g3$) that is most similar (distance 1.4 between the items of the pair). Merge $g2$ with $g3$ to form the first cluster. Combine these two genes into a 'protogene' by listing the pairs of sample points (by, for instance, taking the average of each pair of sample points), and then recalculate all pairwise comparisons for the remaining genes, and so on, until all the genes are clustered. So, for instance, the average for the protogene of $g2$ and $g3$ would be (2.5, 1, 0, 1.5), which is the average between the pairs of points ((2,3), (1,1), (0,0), (1,2)). For the second iteration:

$$d(g1, g5) = 5.1 \quad d(g4, g5) = 3.742$$
$$d(g1, g4) = 2.83$$

These are the same as before. Comparing $g1$, $g4$ and $g5$ with the new protogene gives:

$$d(g1, g_{2,3}) = \sqrt{(3 - 2.5)^2 + (2 - 1)^2 + (1 - 0)^2 + (1 - 1.5)^2}$$
$$= \sqrt{0.25 + 1 + 1 + 0.25}$$
$$= 1.58$$
$$d(g4, g_{2,3}) = \sqrt{(1 - 2.5)^2 + (0 - 1)^2 + (1 - 0)^2 + (0 - 1.5)^2}$$
$$= \sqrt{2.25 + 1 + 1 + 2.25}$$
$$= 2.55$$
$$d(g5, g_{2,3}) = \sqrt{(0 - 2.5)^2 + (0 - 1)^2 + (3 - 0)^2 + (3 - 1.5)^2}$$
$$= \sqrt{6.25 + 1 + 9 + 2.25}$$
$$= 4.3$$

The most similar pair at the end of the second iteration is $g1$ with $g_{2,3}$ (with value 1.58). This becomes a new protogene, with new averages calculated for this protogene *either* by adding the values of all three genes for each sample together and dividing by three (e.g. for patient 1, g_1 value of 3, g_2 value of 2, and g_3 value of 3, giving average 2.67), *or* by treating the $g_{2,3}$ as one gene and calculating a new average based on just two sample values (e.g. for patient 1, $g_{2,3}$ value of 2.5 and g_1 value of 3, giving average 2.75). Adopt the latter strategy, giving a new protogene $g_{1,2,3}$ with values 2.75, 1.5, 0.5 and 0.75 for the four patients, respectively.

The third iteration will consist of pairwise comparisons between gene 4, gene 5 and the new protogene:

$$d(g4, g5) = 3.742$$
$$d(g4, g_{1,2,3}) = \sqrt{(1 - 2.75)^2 + (0 - 1.5)^2 + (1 - 0.5)^2 + (0 - 0.75)^2}$$
$$= \sqrt{3.06 + 2.25 + 0.25 + 0.56} = 2.47$$
$$d(g5, g_{1,2,3}) = \sqrt{(0 - 2.75)^2 + (0 - 1.5)^2 + (3 - 0.5)^2 + (3 - 0.75)^2}$$
$$= \sqrt{7.56 + 2.25 + 6.25 + 5.06} = 4.6.$$

The most similar pair now is $g4$ with $g_{1,2,3}$. This gives a new protogene $g_{1,2,3,4}$ with values 0.5, 0, 2 and 1.5. The final step is to compare the two protogenes $g_{1,2,3,4}$ and $g5$:

$$d(g_{1,2,3,4}, g5) = \sqrt{(0.5 - 0)^2 + (0 - 0)^2 + (2 - 3)^2 + (1.5 - 3)^2}$$
$$= \sqrt{0.25 + 0 + 1 + 2.25} = 1.87.$$

Putting all this together, the gene clustering diagram in Figure 5.4(a) is obtained, where the patient values are described in the order $p1, p2, p3$ and $p4$. But patient samples can also be clustered. Applying the Euclidean method for clustering patients to a transposed version of Table 5.4 (Table 5.5), the first iteration is:

$$d(p1, p2) = \sqrt{(3-2)^2 + (2-1)^2 + (3-1)^2 + (1-0)^2 + (0-0)^2} = 2.65$$
$$d(p1, p3) = 5.1$$
$$d(p1, p4) = 4.58$$
$$d(p2, p3) = 3.61$$
$$d(p2, p4) = 3.74$$
$$d(p3, p4) = 2.65.$$

Table 5.5 The transposed version of the data in Table 5.4, in preparation for patient clustering

	Gene 1	Gene 2	Gene 3	Gene 4	Gene 5
Patient 1	3	2	3	1	0
Patient 2	2	1	1	0	0
Patient 3	1	0	0	1	3
Patient 4	0	1	2	0	3

There are two clusters of $p1$ with $p2$, and $p3$ with $p4$ with value 2.65. Form 'superpatients' from each of these and calculate the new means: $p_{1,2} = (2.5, 1.5, 2, 0.5, 0)$ and $p_{3,4} = (0.5, 0.5, 1, 0.5, 0)$. These two superpatients have similarity:

$$d(p_{1,2}, p_{3,4}) =$$
$$\sqrt{(2.5-0.5)^2 + (1.5-0.5)^2 + (2-1)^2 + (0.5-0.5)^2 + (0-0)^2} = 2.45$$

The final clusterings for both genes and patients are provided in Figure 5.4(b).

If $p3$ and $p4$ belong to one particular class, such as being prostate cancer sufferers, whereas $p1$ and $p2$ belong to another class, such as normal, the clusterings in Figure 5.4(b) would indicate that Gene 5 separates $p3$ and $p4$ as a pair from $p1$ and $p2$, and that Gene 1 and Gene 4 further separate $p3$ from $p4$ (perhaps severity of the cancer).

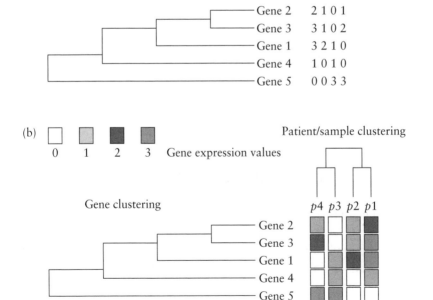

Figure 5.4 (a) Represents the results of clustering just the genes, whereas (b) represents the results of clustering the samples as well. Also, each gene expression value has been given a different shade so that a visual representation of gene clustering is obtained

A number of methods exist for forming clusters in addition to those described above, which is a form of hierarchical cluster method that requires each sample or gene to form its own unique point in space, with successive iterations used to merge two samples into a cluster and then clusters into 'superclusters' depending on their distance from each other. Other clustering methods first allocate each sample or point uniquely to a cluster so that several clusters exist after the first round of iterations. Clusters are then linked together by using a pair of points, one from each cluster, which is closest to each other ('single linkage clustering') or furthest from each other ('total linkage clustering'), rather than adopting a hierarchical approach as in this chapter.

The importance of clustering gene expression data was demonstrated by Eisen *et al.* (1998) when they analysed gene expression of the *Saccharomyces cerevisiae* during the diauxic shift, mitotic cell division cycle, sporulation, and temperature and reducing shocks. The data consisted of all genes for which functional annotation was available (2467). They applied hierarchical clustering using the average linkage method, using averages for the joined elements as they formed the tree. Their analysis clearly demonstrated that genes of similar function cluster together and that groups of coexpressed genes are involved in common cellular processes. Genes of unrelated sequence but similar function were also found to be clustered together. The software used by Eisen *et al.* is available publicly as 'Cluster' and 'Treeview' (for Windows only) and can be downloaded from http://rana.lbl.gov/EisenSoftware.htm. Images produced by these two pieces of software are among the most common seen in gene expression analysis.

5.6 Application guidelines

Nearest neighbour and clustering approaches to data analysis are some of the oldest described in this book. As such, they have found a huge number of applications in academia and industry ranging from the sciences and engineering to more abstract problems. In addition to their longevity, each of these techniques benefits from simplicity. For the most basic techniques, a nearest neighbour or clustering approach can be implemented very easily, as the algorithms themselves are simple and can be applied directly to the data. There are few complex transformations to be done. A good reference here is Sami Kaski's web page http://www.cis.hut.fi/~sami/thesis/node2.html. It comes as no surprise that bioinformatics has also made full use of these techniques in the short time that it has existed. Clustering techniques in particular are probably one of the most well used techniques in problem areas where the data has high-dimensionality (for instance in gene expression analysis). They can be used in their own right to determine useful information from high-dimensional data, but also as a method for pre-processing data for use by other algorithms which benefit from the lower number of variables. Essentially, if similarities between variables of the data are required from an algorithm, clustering techniques provide this with little computational effort. The Bioinformatics Toolbox from http://www.mathworks.com provides a useful set of clustering algorithms for Matlab. Yeung, Medvedovic and Bumgarner (2003) apply clustering to repeated measurement gene expression data, and the software they used can be downloaded from http://expression.microslu.washington.edu/expression/kayee/cluster 2003/yeunggb2003.html. More complex relationships and structures which involve interactions between variables often require the use of other techniques. Similarly, nearest neighbour techniques can provide a fast and computationally efficient method for classifying new data, but are generally not as accurate as some other classification techniques seen here. Both algorithms could provide good solutions where implementation and computation time are a priority.

Almost all bioinformatics websites and journals have sections regarding clustering as it is probably the most ubiquitous technique in bioinformatics applications. Therefore no single resource is recommended for this: inputting the keywords 'clustering' and 'bioinformatics' into a search engine such as Google[2] (or more specifically Citeseer[3]) will yield a large number of resources.

5.7 Summary of chapter

1   Nearest neighbour and clustering approaches are examples of 'unsupervised' techniques in that they attempt to find relationships among attributes and samples by using only patterns of coexpression and similarity among attribute values shared by samples.

2   Unsupervised gene expression data analysis consists of expression profile clustering to find groups of coexpressed genes in static data

---

[2] See http://www.google.com.
[3] See http://www.citeseer.com.

(that is, data that is not measured over time) or, if temporal gene expression data is available, coregulated genes (that is, genes that are all expressed or not expressed together at certain time points).

3   Unsupervised approaches do not rely on additional information, such as the class into which a sample falls, to build their clusterings.

4   Unsupervised approaches are therefore considered 'natural' by many researchers in that they find natural partitions of samples and/or genes into subsets.

5   However, there are a number of problems with clustering, including different results being returned depending on the clustering methods adopted (which means that researchers need to know something about the techniques used) and interpretation of the final cluster diagrams.

6   Nevertheless, clustering is useful for identifying genes that are maximally differentiated from each other for further analysis as to their possible roles in partitioning samples.

5.8 References

Dasarathy, B.V. (1991) *Nearest Neighbor (NN) Norms: NN Pattern Classification Techniques*. IEEE Computer Society Press.

Eisen, M.B., Spellman, P.T., Brown, P.O. *et al*. (1998) Cluster analysis and display of genome-wide expression patterns. *Proc. Natl. Acad. Sci.*, **95**, 14863–14868.

Friedman, J.H., Bentley, J.L. and Raphael, A.F. (1977) An algorithm for finding best matches in logarithmic expected time. *ACM Transactions on Mathematical Software*, 3(3), 209–226.

Levin, J. (1997) Exploring the limits of nearest neighbour secondary structure prediction. *Protein Eng.*, **7**, 771–776.

Levin, J., Robson, B. and Garner, J. (1986) An algorithm for secondary structure determination in proteins based on sequence similarity. *FEBS*, **205**, 303–308.

Michener, C.D., and Sokal, R.R. (1957) A quantitative approach to a problem in classification. *Evolution*, **11**, 130–162.

Sneath, P. H. A. and Sokal, R.R. (1973) *Numerical Taxonomy*. Freeman, San Francisco.

Winston, P.H. (1992) *Artificial Intelligence*. Addison Wesley.

Yeung, K.Y., Medvedovic, M. and Bumgarner, R.E. (2003) Clustering gene-expression data with repeated measurements. *Genome Biology*, 4:R34 (Open access: http://genomebiology.com/2003/4/5/R34).

6

Identification (Decision) Trees

6.1 Method

Identification trees are probably the most widely applied intelligent technique. They have been used for a huge variety of applications in commerce and academia ranging from the sciences, through engineering to financial, commercial and risk-based applications. In fact, identification trees are most used in everyday life as they are often applied in the retail sector where they are used to determine and predict our shopping and spending habits. Practically every store has a loyalty scheme of some description, and the terabytes of data that are collected about customers contain salient information about how and why we behave in the way that we do. To discover this information from the data, it must be mined to reveal the interesting features and remove those that are irrelevant or noisy. It is in this process of data mining that identification trees have become most well known. Their success in these commercial areas can also benefit the field of bioinformatics as many problems in this field consist of large amounts of noisy data. As with many techniques, the success of the identification tree approach is due partly to its simplicity and efficiency. In terms of its execution, the identification tree is an algorithm that has few complex steps. The following section describes the notion of classification and the method that the identification tree uses to classify data taken from many domains, including those with very large databases such as bioinformatics.

Intelligent Bioinformatics   Edward Keedwell and Ajit Narayanan
© 2005 John Wiley & Sons, Ltd

Classification

The task of classification is one that is prominent in a large number of application areas. It is essentially the task of creating rules or structures that will group individuals into predetermined classes by identifying common patterns or traits for those individuals, as given by the data. The identification tree approach is therefore 'supervised' in that the algorithm has knowledge of the classes into which individuals fall when constructing rules or structures for classification. This is to be contrasted with the 'unsupervised' approaches of Chapter 5, where nearest neighbour and clustering techniques partition the data into subsets depending on similar patterns of values across the attributes of the dataset. Classification can be used to answer a wide variety of questions in many application areas. For instance, questions that can potentially be answered by employing classification include the following.

1   What features make an individual prone to sunburn?

2   What features of a Post Office make it more or less prone to robbery or burglary?

3   What are the genetic differences between diseased individuals and normal individuals?

In each of these examples, at least two, mutually exclusive classes are required (e.g. 'sunburnt' versus 'non-sunburnt'; 'high-risk' versus 'medium risk' versus 'low risk'; 'diseased' versus 'normal') into which all samples fall, where these classes are predetermined and included in the data. The task for the classification algorithm is to select, across a dataset of individuals or samples with known class, those features (or attributes, or variables) which are most strongly associated with a particular classification for each sample. Normally there is no restriction to the number of features that are used, but classification algorithms are compared on their accuracy and the number of features used for classifying all samples. The fewer the number of features used for classifying all samples therefore, the better the solution. The goal of classification algorithms is to produce a rule set (called a 'classification model') that uses the fewest number of attributes/features for classifying all the samples in the database, on the assumption that these attributes/features are the most important for classification. Compact solutions are important because the results of the classification process often have to be scrutinized by individuals who are experts in their domain, and complex solutions involving a large number of features are often very difficult to interpret.

This ability to interpret and evaluate a classification model is perhaps even more important in bioinformatics, as often the bioinformatician is not an expert in the biological or biomedical field in question. Small and accurate solutions to classification problems are the most desired, and the identification tree algorithm has built its reputation on discovering these in other domains.

Identification trees

Identification trees have proved very successful in the classification domain for a number of reasons.

1 They are relatively undemanding in computational terms in comparison with other techniques in this book.

2 They provide clear, explicit reasoning of their decision making in the form of symbolic decision trees which can be converted to sets of rules.

3 They are accurate and, in more recent guises, increasingly robust in the face of noise.

Identification trees, as their name suggests, produce a tree of features that provide tests for classifying each of the samples/records in the data according to their most salient features. The basic premise is that only a few features are required to classify all the samples, and the problem for a classification algorithm is to search for and identify this reduced feature set given all the features in the dataset. The approach is to test each feature iteratively to identify its potential for dividing the samples so that they fall into the given classes. This is best shown with an example.

Table 6.1 shows some example data about the umpires' decision to play a cricket match. As cricket is played outside, there are various factors that determine whether the umpires will allow play to take place. In this example, data on three factors thought to be influencing the decision, namely the weather, the light and the condition of the ground, is collected and stored.

Table 6.1　Factors influencing the umpires' decision to play a cricket match

Weather	Light	Ground condition	Umpires' decision
Sunny	Good	Dry	Play
Overcast	Good	Dry	Play
Raining	Good	Dry	No play
Overcast	Poor	Dry	No play
Overcast	Poor	Damp	No play
Raining	Poor	Damp	No play
Overcast	Good	Damp	Play
Sunny	Poor	Dry	Play

From this data, an identification tree can be constructed that can show which are the important factors in making the decision. It is obvious that there is not one feature that can determine whether play will take place (classify the dataset completely).The task is to determine, from the data, the rules the umpires are explicitly or implicitly using to determine whether play should take place. An identification tree can be constructed which will provide information as to which features are important in making the decision.

Identification tree algorithm summary

The aim of the identification tree algorithm is to split the data so that each subset of the data uniquely identifies a class in the data. Some of the terms in this summary may not be familiar, but are explained in the detailed algorithm description. The decision tree algorithm can simply be summarized as follows.

1　For each feature, compute the *gain criterion.*

2　Select the best feature and split the data according to the values in that feature.

3　If each of the subsets contains just one class then stop. Otherwise, reapply points 1–3 on each of the subsets of data.

4　If the data is not completely classified but there are no more splits available then stop.

Identification tree algorithm detail

The algorithm needs to divide up the set of training examples into two smaller sets that completely encapsulate each class 'Play' and 'No play'. The 'supervised' aspects of the algorithm in contrast to the unsupervised techniques of the previous chapter, consist of the class values being used to determine the effectiveness of an attribute in being able to partition the samples consistently into one of these classes. Each division is known as a test and splits the dataset in subsets according to the value of the feature. For instance if a test on 'Light' is performed this gives:

Light = Good: yields four examples, three of class 'Play' and one of 'No play'

Sunny	Good	Dry	Play
Overcast	Good	Dry	Play
Overcast	Good	Damp	Play
Raining	Good	Dry	No play

Light = Poor: yields four examples, one of class 'No play' and three of 'Play'

Overcast	Poor	Dry	No play
Overcast	Poor	Damp	No play
Sunny	Poor	Dry	Play
Raining	Poor	Damp	No play

Notice that no attention is paid to the other two attributes 'Weather' and 'Ground condition' when testing the effectiveness of 'Light'. The above test on 'Light' separates the samples into two subsets, each with three examples of one class and one of another. In a different problem, this might be considered a good result, and it would be true that the light level would have an impact on whether the umpires allowed play to take place. In this example, this test has been chosen at random and is not the best way of splitting the data. Therefore a measurement of the effectiveness of each attribute/feature is required by the algorithm to determine which feature is best for classifying the samples. This measure must reflect the distribution of examples over the classes in the problem. The best-known currently employed measure is known as the gain criterion.

6.2 Gain criterion

The gain criterion is based on the amount of information that a test on the data conveys. This information-theory based approach has been shown to be more effective than a simple tally of the number of individuals in each class, and is the primary method used in commercial packages including See5 and C4.5.[1] The information contained within a test is related to the probability of selecting one training example from that class. This probability is easily described by noting the frequency with which a particular class C_j appears in the training set T:

$$\frac{freq(C_j, T)}{|T|}. \tag{6.1}$$

The information conveyed by this is then computed as $-\log_2$ of the probability. This gives:

$$-\log_2\left(\frac{freq(C_j, T)}{|T|}\right). \tag{6.2}$$

This equation therefore computes the information conveyed from each class of the training set and to get the expected information from the training set as a whole, this measure is summed over all classes, multiplying by their relative frequencies:

$$in(T) = -\sum_{j=1}^{k} \frac{freq(C_j, T)}{|T|} * \log_2\left(\frac{freq(C_j, T)}{|T|}\right). \tag{6.3}$$

This gives the information measure for the entire training set. Each test that is devised by the algorithm must be compared with this to determine how much of an improvement (if any) is seen in classification. When a test is performed, the data is split into a number of new subsets (as seen previously when the data was split using 'Light'). To measure the information yielded by a split x the weighted sum over the subsets is used:

$$in_x(T) = -\sum_{i=1}^{n} \frac{|T_i|}{|T|} * \log_2\left(\frac{freq(C_j, T)}{|T|}\right). \tag{6.4}$$

The gain given by a particular test can be given by subtracting the result of Equation 6.4 from Equation 6.3:

$$gain(X) = in(T) - in_x(T). \tag{6.5}$$

---

[1] This software and documentation is available from http://www.rulequest.com.

The identification tree algorithm proceeds through each feature, computing the gain criterion for each feature, selects the best of these, and then uses the same method on the remaining subsets.

This can be seen more clearly in the example given above. First, the decision tree will evaluate all possible features. We start with the hypothesis that no features are important and then check each of the features in turn:

$$in(T) = -4/8 * \log_2(4/8) - 4/8 * \log_2(4/8) = 1.0$$

$$
\begin{aligned}
in_{\text{weather}}(T) = \; & 2/8 * (-2/2 * \log_2(2/2) - 0/2 * \log_2(0/2)) && \text{(Sunny)} \\
& + 4/8 * (-2/4 * \log_2(2/4) - 2/4 * \log_2(2/4)) && \text{(Overcast)} \\
& + 2/8 * (-0/2 * \log_2(0/2) - 2/2 * \log_2(2/2)) && \text{(Raining)} \\
& = 0.5 \text{ bits.} \\
& \textbf{Gain} = 1.0 - 0.5 = 0.5. \\
in_{\text{light}}(T) = \; & 4/8 * (-3/4 * \log_2(3/4) - 1/4 * \log_2(1/4)) && \text{(Good)} \\
& + 4/8 * (-1/4 * \log_2(1/4) - 3/4 * \log_2(3/4)) && \text{(Poor)} \\
& = 0.811 \text{ bits.} \\
& \textbf{Gain} = 1.0 - 0.811 = 0.189. \\
in_{\text{ground}}(T) = \; & 5/8 * (-3/5 * \log_2(3/5) - 2/5 * \log_2(2/5)) && \text{(Dry)} \\
& + 3/8 * (-1/3 * \log_2(1/3) - 2/3 * \log_2(2/3)) && \text{(Damp)} \\
& = 0.951 \text{ bits.} \\
& \textbf{Gain} = 1.0 - 0.951 = 0.049.
\end{aligned}
$$

For instance, for 'weather', two of the eight samples (2/8) have the attribute value 'Sunny', of which two out of two (2/2) fall in the class 'Play' (the first and eighth samples in Table 6.1) and none of the two (0/2) fall in the class 'No play', plus (+) four out of eight samples have the attribute value 'Overcast', of which two out of four (2/4) fall in the class 'Play' and two out of four (2/4) fall in the class 'No play', plus (+) two out of eight (2/8) samples have the attribute 'Raining', of which none of the two (0/2) fall in the class 'Play' and two out of two (2/2) fall in the class 'No play'. In this example, the feature 'Weather' would be selected as the first attribute on which to split the data as it has a far higher information gain (0.5) compared with the other two features (0.189 and 0.049). This constitutes the first node of the tree and now the training data is split into three sets, one each for 'Sunny' 'Overcast' and 'Raining'. Two of these three sets (those for 'Sunny' and 'Raining') have individuals of only one class ('Play' and 'No play', respectively), so no further action is required on them. However the 'Overcast' subset has two individuals of class 'Play' and two of 'No play'. The algorithm now proceeds to investigate whether a further test using one of the remaining two features can classify this dataset correctly.

Weather	Light	Ground condition	Umpires' decision
Overcast	Good	Dry	Play
Overcast	Poor	Dry	No play
Overcast	Poor	Damp	No play
Overcast	Good	Damp	Play

By considering the remaining data as a new sample set (S), the same procedure can be used to determine a new split to improve the current tree:

$$in(S) = \quad -2/4 * \log_2(2/4) - 2/4 * \log_2(2/4) = 1.0 \text{ bits.}$$

$$
\begin{aligned}
in_{\text{light}}(S) = \quad & 2/4 * (-2/2 * \log_2(0/2) - 0/2 * \log_2(0/2)) && \text{(Good)} \\
& +2/4 * (-0/2 * \log_2(0/2) - 2/2 * \log_2(2/2)) && \text{(Poor)} \\
& = 0.0 \text{ bits.} \\
& \textbf{Gain} = 1.0 - 0.0 = 1.0.
\end{aligned}
$$

$$
\begin{aligned}
in_{\text{ground}}(S) = \quad & 2/4 * (-1/2 * \log_2(1/2) - 1/2 * \log_2(1/2)) && \text{(Dry)} \\
& +2/4 * (-1/2 * log_2(1/2) - -1/2 * log_2(1/2)) && \text{(Damp)} \\
& = 1.0 \text{ bits.} \\
& \textbf{Gain} = 1.0 - 1.0 = 0.0.
\end{aligned}
$$

In this second iteration the algorithm has found that by splitting this subset of data on the feature 'Light', the data is completely classified. That is, each subset of the data as determined by the decision tree has only individuals belonging to one class in the set. The final decision tree can be seen in Figure 6.1.

The construction of the tree is reasonably simple, as the same computation can be applied to the increasingly small sets of data as determined by previous splits. This algorithm therefore represents an elegant solution to the problem of supervised classification in datasets.

Continuous data

The example above uses only discrete data, where each feature is split up into a number of categories that are used in the decision tree. Real-world – and especially biological – data contain a lot of continuous (real

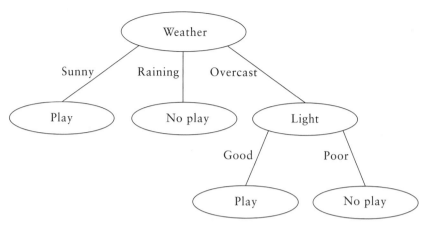

Figure 6.1 The final tree generated by executing the identification tree algorithm on the cricket example dataset; this tree classifies the training data exactly, with two examples at each of the four leaves

or floating point) values and the identification tree algorithm has a system for dealing with these values. The system relies on the fact that whilst the range of the data itself might be continuous in nature, the data presented to the algorithm must, by definition be a set of finite, discrete observations of that continuous range. The continuous data is treated in much the same way as the discrete data, but with one important difference. Whereas the discrete data uses the '=' operator, the continuous data uses the comparison operators ('<', '≤', '>', '≥') to determine the subsets of the data created by a test. There are $n - 1$ possible tests given a continuous attribute which has n possible values, but generally speaking the evaluation of each of these tests can be determined in short computational time. It is in this fashion that the decision tree algorithm can be used for classification with continuous and discrete values.

For instance, if the 'Light' attribute had contained values ranging from '1' (very poor light) to 10 ('excellent light'), one test resulting from the identification tree algorithm might be 'If Light ≥ 6 then Play', which would return a figure describing how many Play cases with a value of 6 or more for the 'Light' attribute are captured by this test. The identification tree algorithm can test different continuous values in the range of values for an attribute for their effect on classification and choose appropriate thresholds to maximize the correct number of cases falling on either side of the comparison tests.

Gain ratio

The gain ratio seen in Quinlan (1993) is a more sophisticated version of its forerunner, the gain criterion. The difficulty with the gain criterion is that it is biased towards tests which have many subsets. For instance, the split on 'weather' produced a dataset with three subsets, one each for overcast, sunny and raining. The remaining two attributes ('light' and 'ground') yielded two subsets. We will see in the following example, the gain criterion weighted the split on 'weather' more favourably than it should have because of the larger number of values the attribute has. This behaviour is to be avoided as tests that result in many subsets are not necessarily those that will yield the most useful information. The gain ratio (Quinlan, 1993) is a revised gain measure that takes into account the size of the subsets created by test. To compute the gain ratio, the gain (as computed in Equation 6.5) is divided by the information contained by the number of subsets in the split. This 'split information' measure can be used to normalize the gain criterion seen above, and is computed as:

$$splitin(X) = -\sum_{i=1}^{n} \frac{|T_i|}{|T|} * \log_2 \left(\frac{|T_i|}{|T|} \right). \qquad (6.6)$$

This gives a final gain ratio equation:

$$gainratio(X) = \frac{gain(X)}{splitin(X)}. \qquad (6.7)$$

Returning to the example above, if the data is split on the attribute 'weather' then three subsets are created, two of which contain two records, and one which contains four. The split information can therefore be computed as:

$$-2/8 * \log_2(2/8) - 2/8 * \log_2(2/8) - 4/8 * \log_2(4/8) = 1.5$$

Taking the gain criterion score of 0.5 for the attribute 'weather' from the example above, the gain ratio is computed as:

$$0.5/1.5 = 0.33.$$

Splits on the other attributes in the data yield two even subsets with four records apiece in them, which yields a split information of 1.0. In this circumstance, the gain criterion values remain unchanged for attributes 'light' and 'ground condition', and the attribute 'weather' is still chosen as the first split in the tree. However, its influence has been reduced (from 0.5 using gain criterion to 0.33 using gain ratio) so the effect on the gain criterion exerted by the fact that the attribute splits the data into more subsets has been reduced somewhat by using the gain ratio.

By using a simple algorithm and an information-theory approach, the identification tree can discover useful and accurate information from a set of data which may not be obvious on first observation. The small example dataset, when combined with the ability to process continuous values and a revised gain ratio, illustrates the principles behind the execution of the identification tree algorithm. These improvements to the algorithm become increasingly valuable when there are thousands or millions of data records in the dataset. With data of this size and type, which is frequently the norm in commercial and scientific applications, a robust, efficient and accurate algorithm is necessary to extract meaning from the collected data. The entire process of data collection, manipulation, knowledge discovery and interpretation is known as data mining and probably constitutes the single largest application of artificial intelligence techniques outside the academic laboratory. The identification tree algorithm is certainly not the only data mining algorithm, but it is one of the most popular. There are, however, some drawbacks to the approach.

6.3 Over fitting and pruning

To a certain extent every algorithm involved with classification runs the risk of over fitting the data. This is the phenomenon where the algorithm learns the errors (noise) in the data as well as the underlying structure of the processes that created the data. This phenomenon occurs because every algorithm attempts to reduce the error in classifying the data, and many algorithms including identification trees can reduce this error by introducing more and more splits in the data. When this happens the model can become overly complex, which in itself is not desirable due to the increase in model size, and therefore it cannot be interpreted as easily. However, a further effect is that the tree becomes so accurate on the training data samples that a new sample not seen previously by the identification tree is falsely classified. Essentially, the algorithm has learnt the training data *too well* in that it has learnt the erroneous data as well as the underlying patterns. To identify when this problem occurs, the data can be divided into two sets: the training set and the test set. The training set usually comprises about 75 per cent of the total dataset, with the remaining 25 per cent of samples kept back precisely to check on overfitting. The identification tree algorithm is then 'trained' on the training set only, and when it has constructed a tree the test set is fed to the tree to check on the accuracy of the tree. The class into which each of the samples in the test set falls is of course known, and this knowledge can be used to check on the accuracy of the identification tree. A variant of this method is to run this 'train–test' regime on several different training and test sets randomly generated from the original data. Providing that the test data has been drawn from the same population as the training, then this deleterious effect can be determined as overfitting and a strategy should be used to overcome it.

A widely-used strategy for dealing with over fitting is pruning. This is a process whereby the entire tree is generated as previously described until no more good splits can be made. Once this has occurred, the tree is pruned back, according to certain criteria, so that complex branches of the tree are consolidated into smaller, perhaps less accurate (on the training data) sub-branches. This is obviously less efficient than simply generating a smaller tree in the first place, but Quinlan (1993) states that the method of generating and pruning performs more reliably than stopping or prepruning. Any subtree (that is not a leaf) can be considered for reduction to a leaf where the leaf classification is the most frequent class member of that subtree. However, the pruning method must use some estimate of the expected error of:

1   the current subtree, and

2   the leaf that is replacing the current subtree.

If restricted to the training data, the current subtree will have the fewest errors every time, so some measure must be made of the expected error incurred on other data. This can either be done by using data set aside for testing (although as this data will be used to tune the model, a further 'test' set will be required to truly evaluate performance at a later stage), or by using some heuristic estimate. Quinlan (1993) uses a heuristic based on the upper bound of the binomial distribution, due to the fact that often (and especially in bioinformatics problems) there is not enough data to generate one or more hold-out sets for testing. The concept of pruning is included here because the level of pruning is often a parameter in constructing an identification tree and can influence the accuracy of the results that are obtained. In addition to this, it is important to note that a complete decision tree is seldom kept in its unpruned form and some level of pruning is required for the tree to generalize beyond its training set.

Other disadvantages with identification trees

Whilst the simplicity and efficiency of the identification tree algorithm is central to its popularity, this approach has also been criticized in some quarters. The majority of the criticism focuses on the deterministic way the algorithm splits the data. The example seen previously shows the algorithm selected the first split on the attribute 'Weather'. However, it may be that by splitting the data firstly by weather, that other effects in the data are lost. The fact that the split in the data is selected based on the fact that it has the best gain criterion at a certain stage is a central tenet of the approach and is instrumental in its efficiency. However, the approach would benefit from some element of depth-first search where the split is evaluated not only on its current ability to classify the data, but the accuracy of the split later on in the algorithm run. Inevitably, this would lead to a greatly increased amount of computation, as a partial or even entire tree would have to be generated for each split and there may only be a small number of problems which would benefit from its application. The tree-like nature of the identification trees ensures that the first split will always be the most important, but it is only evaluated as to how well it classifies the data at that particular point. It may be that another tree exists, with a different starting split, which classifies the data much more accurately. There have been a number of methods suggested to counteract this effect, including the use of other algorithms to select the starting split for the decision tree (this approach is seen in one of the applications later in this chapter). However, these approaches are liable to require more computation than the original algorithm and therefore may not be as amenable to large datasets.

Conclusions

Identification trees have been used extensively in industry and academia and are perhaps the most widely applied artificial intelligence technique covered in this book. This success is largely attributable to the efficiency of the algorithm which enables it to be applied to huge datasets that other algorithms could not mine within a reasonable time scale. With businesses collecting terabytes of data relating to customer transactions and other business activity, this efficiency is vital and, as is often the case, is due largely to the simplicity of the approach. This efficiency is in turn due to the simplicity of the split evaluation function, based on information-theory approaches; it does not require any complex mathematics to develop a highly accurate assessment of the effectiveness of a split. For bioinformatics, though, it remains to be seen whether identification tree approaches will become as prevalent as they are in other domains. Bioinformatics data (such as gene expression data) often has a vast number of variables (genes), but a small number of records (experiments) in contrast to commercial data which is often the reverse of this and so algorithms must be efficient given this atypical level of complexity.

6.4 Application guidelines

Introduction

Identification trees as described previously can be used in a large variety of situations where information is required from a set of data collected from a variety of sources. They are especially useful when there are a large number of records in the data. In addition to this, they can be used when explicit reasons for classification need to be provided, for instance in applications where safety-critical considerations prevail or where the results need to be scrutinized by expert users. This is often the case in bioinformatics problems where the results need to be tested by biologists to determine whether the results have biological plausibility.

Therefore, when the results are required to be explicit and when there is a lot of data, identification trees can discover knowledge in good time. However, they are essentially restricted to problems of classification where the class of the training set individuals is known. As such, they cannot be considered as flexible as some of the other techniques in this book such as genetic algorithms, genetic programming or neural networks, as these techniques can be used for a variety of purposes, in addition to classification. This supervised approach is in contrast to the other 'unsupervised' techniques seen in this book such as clustering

(Chapter 5) and kohonen networks (Chapter 7) which do not require this explicit definition of class within the data.

Cross-validation

An important aspect of applying any machine learning technique to bioinformatics problems, but especially identification trees, is the use of test data. Often in bioinformatics problems the number of data records available for an experiment (especially in the case of microarray experiments) can be small relative to the number of attributes. Therefore it may not be feasible to split the data into separate large training and test sets. Instead, cross-validation can be used where the algorithm is run repeatedly on different training and test sets. Cross-validation splits the entire dataset into a number of folds, which is determined by the experimenter and the amount of data available. If the data is split into five folds, then the machine learning technique is trained on four fifths of the data and then tested on the remaining one fifth. This is then repeated for all the other four folds in the dataset, testing on a different fold each time. The measure of accuracy is determined by the average error of each run on each fold of the dataset. Figure 6.2 shows this process graphically. In this example, the training dataset is split into eight sections, seven of which are combined and used to train the identification tree and the remaining fold used to test the example. This is repeated for the N (in this case eight) folds in the dataset and the average accuracy or error reported over the N runs of the algorithm. One advantage of this approach is that, at the end of the five-fold process, there will be five possibly different identification trees. Future samples with unknown class can then be fed to all five identification trees and a 'majority vote' taken as to which class the new sample falls into.

As described previously, the number of folds chosen is usually determined by the computational time available to the experimenter (more folds take more time to run) and the amount of data in the dataset. A popular specific cross-validation technique is 'leave-one-out' cross-validation which, as its name suggests, leaves one example out of the dataset for testing and trains the algorithm on the remaining data. This is still N-fold cross-validation, but where N is equal to the number of data records (individuals or samples) in the dataset, and is the most computationally demanding cross-validation technique as N trials must be run. The cross-validation process gives a good impression of the accuracy of

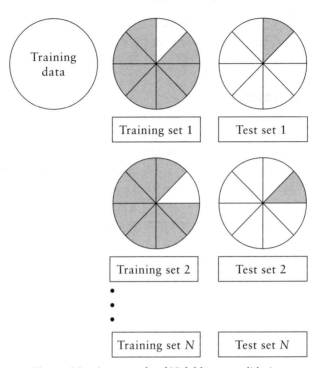

Figure 6.2   An example of N-fold cross-validation

the approach that can be expected on non-training data and is especially useful where the amount of data is restricted, which is often the case in problems in biology.

Software

Data mining is big business and identification tree software forms a reasonably large sector of this market, so there are various implementations to choose from. However, because they are used so frequently by large corporations, the larger packages can often be costly. These packages tend to incorporate a large amount of external software which allows connection to a variety of databases, exporting results in a number of formats and good visualization of the results. If these extra features are required, the SPSS Clementine[2] package is frequently described as the industry standard and includes a number of approaches (neural networks, nearest neighbour algorithms and, of course, identification trees)

---

[2] More information can be found at http://www.spss.com/clementine.

described in this book. If a more cut-down identification tree software package is required, then See5 (Windows) or C5 (UNIX)[3], developed by Ross Quinlan, represents a neat and efficient implementation of the algorithms discussed here. In addition to this, See5 is kept up-to-date with the latest advances in the field so that it incorporates new features such as 'boosting', 'cross-validation' and 'fuzzy thresholds'. If a simple and quick algorithm implementation is required with rudimentary visualization of results, then See5 is highly recommended. An alternative to this package is CART[4] (Breiman *et al.*, 1984) which should be considered when choosing a decision tree algorithm.

As might be expected for a technique that was conceived up to 20 years ago, there are a number of open source sites with code for identification tree algorithms. An excellent public-domain library of machine learning code written by Ron Kohavi is available from SGI[5]. This includes a large variety of algorithms, including variants of C4.5 (as described above) and other rule induction approaches such as CN2 and is available for both Windows and UNIX operating systems. Written in C++, this is more than a simple implementation of the algorithms since it includes a variety of utilities and is also well documented.

6.5 Bioinformatics applications

HIV and Hepatitis C (HCV) protease cleavage prediction

As previously described in Chapter 2, viral protease is one of the enzymes typically accompanying HIV RNA and HCV into the cell (see Figure 2.10, Chapter 2). It cleaves the precursor viral polyproteins (the substrate) at specific cleavage-recognition sites when they emerge from the ribosomes of the host cell as one long sequence (Figure 6.3(a)). When certain substrate configurations occur (a certain sequence of amino acids), the protease cleaves the viral polyprotein at a specific point in the substrate (Figure 6.3(b)). Conventionally, the polyprotein substrate is labelled with unique P identifiers (one for each amino acid) and the protease region around the active site with unique S identifiers (Figure 6.3(c)).

This cleavage step is essential in the final maturation step of HIV and HCV. That is, protease is responsible for the post-translation processing

---

[3] Available from http://www.rulequest.com.
[4] Available from http://www.salford-systems.com/.
[5] Available from http://www.sgi.com/tech/mlc/index.html.

(a)
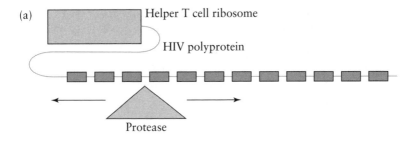

Helper T cell ribosome

HIV polyprotein

Protease

(b)
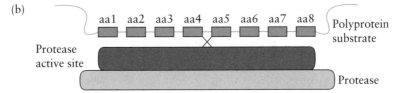

(c)
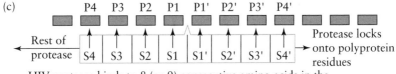

HIV protease binds to 8 (or 9) consecutive amino acids in the
polyprotein before clearing between specific amino acids

(d) Protease inhibition: anti-viral agent consisting of manufacturer pseudo-
polyprotein fragments that 'stick' to the protease through competitive or
non-competitive binding

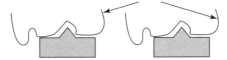

Figure 6.3   The final maturation phase of HIV

of the viral gag and gag-pol polyproteins to yield the structural proteins
and enzymes of the virus for further infection.

There are two current methods for inhibiting viral proteases. Competitive inhibition consists of identifying an inhibitor that will lock on to
the protease's active site and thereby prevent that protease from binding to any further substrate (Figure 6.3(d)). These inhibitors are used
only once (one inhibitor – one protease). Non-competitive inhibition,
on the other hand, works by identifying a regulatory site rather than an
active site of the protease so that the inhibitor, when bound to the regulatory site, distorts the structure of the protease and thereby prevents it

from binding to its substrate. Inhibitors must be carefully and specifically designed so that they do not affect the naturally occurring proteases in the human body.

A significant amount of potential cleavage site data for HIV and HCV has been produced through laboratory *in vitro* experiments, where the effect of these proteases on synthetic oligopeptide sequences have been observed and recorded, constituting data sets for pattern recognition and machine learning applications. Another way to produce negative cleavage sites is to assume that regions between known cleavage sites are non-cleavage. That is, as well as trying to produce cleavage and non-cleavage oligopeptide sequences *in vitro,* the full polyprotein sequence of the virus can be analysed by a computer and fixed length sequences (either eight or 10 amino acids long for the HIV and HCV polyproteins, respectively) which are currently not known to be cleavage sites are extracted as 'negative cleavage' sequences. For HIV, experimental work suggests that cleavage takes place in the middle of an octopeptide substrate (i.e. between the fourth and fifth amino acid), whereas for HCV the situation is more complicated. In fact HCV has at least three proteases, each of which works on distinct regions of the long S. polypeptide sequence. We focus on the region subject to one of these proteases, NS3. For NS3 there is evidence that cleavage takes place between the sixth and seventh amino acid of a decapeptide substrate. For HIV a 363-substrate dataset was available (Cai and Chou, 1998) consisting of 114 sequences that were clinically reported as cleaved and 249 sequences as non-cleaved. For HCV a special dataset was constructed from the literature consisting of 168 NS3-cleaved sequences (as reported in the clinical literature) and 147 sequences that were derived by moving a 10-amino acid substrate window along the HCV polyprotein sequence so that decapeptide regions not overlapping with known cleavage regions or each other (as far as possible) were identified and tagged as non-cleavage. The samples were represented to See5 (Quinlan, 1993) as an eight-character string of amino acids (using the amino acid alphabet) for HIV samples and as 10-character strings for HCV. Each sample was terminated with a '1' to signify cleavage or '0' to signify non-cleavage. The task for See5 was to determine whether there was a pattern of amino acids in the substrate that could help determine whether the viral protease did or did not cleave (Narayanan, Wu and Zhang, 2002), for the design of possible future protease inhibitors.

So, for instance, one HIV sample for See5 was **G,Q,V,N,Y,E,E,F,1,** where **G** occupied first position of the substrate, **Q** the second position, etc., and the final **1** signified that this sample was cleaved. An example of a HCV sample is **D,L,E,V,V,R,S,T,W,V,0**, where the 10 positions in the substrate are encoded **D** through to **V** and **0** signifies non-cleavage. The datasets were separately analysed by See5, using a 10-fold cross-validation technique. For HIV the final accuracy figure across all 10 folds on test data was 86 per cent, with 25 false negatives (25/248 non-cleavage cases were incorrectly classed as cleavage) and 26 false positives (26/114 cleavage cases were incorrectly classed as non-cleavage). For HCV the accuracy figures for test data were slightly worse but still respectable at 82 per cent, with 27 (27/147) false negatives and 32 (32/168) false positives.

For the total HIV dataset, the following rules were derived by See5 (where '(x/y)' after each rule signifies the number of false classifications). (a) *If position4 is phenylalanine then cleavage* (35/5). (b) *If position4 is leucine then cleavage* (38/9). (c) *If position4 is serine then non-cleavage* (26/1). (d) *If position4 is tyrosine and position5 is proline then cleavage* (32/5). Other minor rules covering fewer cases tended to reflect the importance of positions 4 and 5 (on either side of the cleavage site). However, none of the rules was successful in capturing the majority of cases (114 positive sequences in total). One interesting piece of new knowledge extracted by See5 was the relative importance of position 6 (*If position6 is glutamate then cleavage* (44/8)). Also, the above rules provide evidence that hydrophobic residues phenylalanine and tyrosine are involved in cleavage site prediction (rules (a) and (d)).

For HCV, the following rules were found. (a) *If position6 is cysteine then cleavage* (133/27). (b) *If position6 is threonine and position4 is valine then cleavage* (28/5). (c) *If position6 is cysteine and position7 is serine then cleavage* (100/33). (d) *If position1 is aspartate then cleavage* (122/41). (e) *If position10 is tyrosine then cleavage* (98/22). (f) *If position10 is leucine then cleavage* (70/27). Since this is the first time that HCV substrates have been analysed in this way, these rules represent potential new knowledge of HCV NS3 substrates. Also, for both HIV and HCV substrates See5 has for the most part found the positions on either side of the cleavage site that intuitively are the most important (positions 4 and 5 for HIV, positions 6 and 7 for HCV), although there is nothing in the representation of the samples to See5 that gave it any indication of where the actual cleavage sites were. This provides some evidence that future protease competitive inhibitors for HIV and HCV will have to pay particular attention to these positions of the substrate if inhibitors are to work effectively.

Classification of cancer by using diagnosis data

A good deal of the classification problems in bioinformatics data are related to the problem of determining the clinical diagnosis of an individual based on gene expression data or some other measurement of cellular activity. The application of identification trees to this classification task provides a good introduction to the application of the technique in bioinformatics. However, the work undertaken by Li *et al.* (2003) takes the decision tree process a step further, by using a committee of trees to decide the outcome of the classification task. The reason for this is similar to the problem described earlier, in that identification trees are deterministic and use the top ranked feature every time a split is required. This leads to only one tree being created that may be sub-optimal, whereas a tree with a different starting point may perform better. Therefore Li *et al.* used a committee of trees which are first started on the best performing feature (the optimal, or C4.5 tree), but a tree is then grown from the second-best performing feature, and then the third best, up to a stopping point. The trees can then be converted to rules (for more information on this procedure see Quinlan (1993)) and added together to create a large knowledge base. This knowledge base can then be used to classify the data, including new examples. There are, however, difficulties when using multiple rules for the same individual; for instance, some of the rules may place the individual in a certain class, and other rules may disagree. This conflicting behaviour is resolved by using the coverage statistic (the number of individual records covered by the rule) as a measure of the efficacy of that rule. Therefore the coverage for each rule that fires is summed for each class (similar to a weighted-voting system) and the class with the highest weight is predicted.

Li *et al.* show that they gain excellent results in comparison with See5, including the latest developments such as boosting, on a variety of classification problems taken from the bioinformatics literature. The results, which are based on the cross-validation of datasets, show that, as expected, the committee approach performs better on these problems than the single C4.5 results with boosting or bagging. The first experiment was conducted on ovarian cancer containing 253 mass spectrometry proteomic samples, 91 of which were controls and 162 of which represented ovarian cancer. Each of these samples contained 15 154 features which were the relative amplitudes of the intensities for each molecular mass/charge identity. A 10-fold cross-validation procedure was used to ensure consistency of results. The results showed that the committee approach classified this dataset with no errors, whereas C4.5 incurred 10 errors. A second experiment was conducted which was designed to distinguish between six sub-types of acute lymphoblastic leukaemia (ALL) by using gene expression profiles. The data here consisted of 327 individual samples, each of which was comprised of 12 558 gene expression values. In a 10-fold cross-validation approach the committee approach incurred errors on seven cases in comparison with 23 for C4.5.

Therefore this study highlights the fact that identification trees by themselves can be difficult to apply to large-scale data with few records such as gene expression or proteomic data due to the fact that it will use only one or two features to classify the set. However, the committee approach shows that with repeated application of the identification tree, including the modification of its parameters, a more complete classifier can be created. Whilst the reported accuracy results are good, the increased accuracy is to be expected to a certain degree, as the committee approach means that the performance will only be as bad as the worst tree in the committee. It is also worth noting that the computation required to generate the committee approach is considerably larger than a single run of the identification tree algorithm. Although the number of individuals in gene expression experiments is currently small, in the future it is possible that the approach, if used on large datasets, will require significant extra computation.

Consensus method for secondary protein structure prediction

The prediction of secondary and tertiary protein structure from the underlying amino acid combinations is one of the most pressing problems in bioinformatics. The secondary structure determines how groups of amino acids form sub-structures such as the coil, helix or extended strand. The correct derivation of the secondary structure provides vital information as to the tertiary structure and therefore the function of the protein. There are various methods which can be used to predict secondary structure, including the DSSP approach which uses hydrogen bond patterns as predictors, the DEFINE algorithm which uses the distance between C-alpha atoms, and the P-CURVE method which finds regularities along a helicoidal axis. As might be expected, these disparate approaches do not necessarily agree with each other when given the same problem and this can create problems for researchers. The work by Selbig, Mevissen and Lengauer (1999) develops the decision tree as a method for achieving consensus between these approaches by creating a dataset of predicted structures from a number of prediction methods for the same dataset. The correct structures for each of the protein elements in the training set is known, and this forms the classification for each of the records in the training set. The identification tree therefore creates rules of the form

IF Method1 = Helix AND Method2
= Helix THEN Consensus = Helix

In this way, the identification tree can choose when it is prudent to use certain structure prediction methods and when to use others. This methodology ensures that prediction performance is at worst the same as the best prediction method, and in the best case should perform better than that. The results were reported on two datasets, one consisting of 396 proteins (the CB396 dataset, Cuff and Barton (1999)) and the 11 CASP3 proteins[6]. For each of these datasets, seven prediction methods are combined in the consensus tree, and an 11-fold cross-validation procedure is used to determine the accuracy of each of the techniques. The prediction accuracy of the consensus method is better than any of the single methods for both datasets, but also achieves improved results in comparison with another consensus method, JPRED. The decision tree approach improves on the JPRED method by achieving a marginal accuracy improvement of 72.9 per cent as opposed to 72.6 per cent on the CB396 dataset. On the CASP3 dataset, however, the approach improves on JPRED by 1 per cent as it achieves 76.0 per cent accuracy.

This therefore shows a good example of how the intelligent approach of the decision tree can be used to optimally combine existing standard methods of secondary structure prediction. It also provides a neat example of how modern machine learning algorithms can be combined with established scientific methods based on chemo-biological principles. The result of this union is improved accuracy on this difficult problem in bioinformatics.

6.6 Background

The decision tree methodology described here in the method section is that of C4.5 (See5) written by Quinlan in 1993. This was predicated, however, by ID3, again created by Quinlan, in the early 1980s which

---

[6] Dataset available from http://predictioncenter.llnl.gov/casp3/Casp3.html.

included the basic structure that is employed in C4.5. The original idea Quinlan credits to Hoveland and Hunt and *concept learning systems* which, as many of the notions in this book seem to have been, were created in the 1950s.

Since Quinlan designed C4.5 and See5, there have not been any significant paradigm-shifts in the way that decision tree software works. There has been an explosion in the number of software packages which use identification or decision trees, but the theory behind them remains much the same. Advances have come in the shape of improvements to the way that splits are evaluated, how the results are visualized and additional methods such as *bagging* and *boosting*. These areas have now become an important area for research in data mining with decision trees.

6.7 Summary of chapter

1   Decision trees use information-theory measures to divide a set of training examples into known classes.

2   They are efficient with respect to the size of the data, and can be run on most datasets with a modest machine.

3   The information discovered by decision trees is easily interpreted and can be converted into rules to be digested by non-technical personnel.

4   Their efficiency and transparency aid their application in many commercial domains, but often their inflexible deterministic approach can prevent them from being used in bioinformatics problems.

6.8 References

Breiman, L., Friedman, J., Olshen, R. *et al.* (1984) *Classification and Regression Trees.* Wadsworth International Group, Belmont, CA.

Cai, Y.D. and Chou, K.C. (1998) Artificial neural network model for predicting HIV protease cleavage sites in protein. *Advances in Engineering Software*, **29–2**, 119–128.

Cuff, J.A. and Barton, G.J. (1999) Evaluation and improvement of multiple sequence methods for protein secondary structure prediction. *Proteins Struct. Funct. Genet.*, **34**, 508–519.

Li, J., Liu, H., Ng, S-K. *et al.* (2003) Discovery of significant rules for classifying cancer diagnosis data. *Bioinformatics*, **19**, Suppl 2, 93–102.

Quinlan, J.R. (1993) *C4.5: Programs for Machine Learning*, Morgan Kauffman, San Mateo, California.

Narayanan, A., Wu, X. and Zhang, R.Y. (2002) Mining viral protease data to extract cleavage knowledge. *Bioinformatics*, **18**, Suppl 1, 5–13.

Selbig, J., Mevissen, T. and Lengauer, T. (1999) Decision tree based formation of consensus protein secondary structure prediction. *Bioinformatics*, **15**, 1039–1046.

7

Neural Networks

7.1 Method

Neural networks were originally conceived as computational models of the way in which the human brain works. Like the human brain, they consist of many units (analogous to neurons and sometimes called by the same name) connected to each other by variable strength links (analogous to axons in the brain). These variable strength links are abstract representations of the way that most neurons actually communicate with each other in the brain: through changes in the rate or frequency of electrical or chemical messages. As with a number of the techniques described in this book, this technique has been inspired by the way biological organisms (in particular humans) solve the problems of computation in nature. As mathematical models, they have found a large number of applications in science and commerce, particularly in the area of finance and market prediction. The attraction of neural networks is that they can 'learn' relationships between sets of variables taken from a system. Once trained, the network can then be shown new examples and asked to predict the outcome of the new data based on the previous examples it has learnt. This quality, known as generalization, is the ability to infer the underlying relationships in the data and being able to apply them to new situations and is the staple reason for their use in such a wide variety of contexts. This may sound similar to the method by which humans learn and, to a very limited extent, this is true. A further property which distinguishes this technique from other computational methods is that of 'graceful degradation'. The knowledge learnt is encoded in the

Intelligent Bioinformatics   Edward Keedwell and Ajit Narayanan
© 2005 John Wiley & Sons, Ltd

network as a set of 'weights', the individual strength of these weights determines the behaviour of the network. Should any of these weights or units be removed, the network can still function but with reduced performance, a little like the human brain. This is in contrast to most other computational techniques which cannot function at all if one or more parts of their decision making process is faulty. Neural networks should not, however, be seen as constituting biologically significant models of human brain activity, although some studies are conducted into the simulation of human brain activity (under the umbrella of connectionism) for the purposes of this book, they are merely useful computational tools. Therefore, as computational tools, neural networks represent somewhat of a departure from many of the other techniques in this book which have a more symbolic flavour. They have a step-by-step algorithm of operation, but the resulting neural structure has a little more in common with biology than the other methods described in this book.

Architecture

A neural network consists of interconnected units, often arranged in layers. The configuration of these units is known as the architecture, and can vary widely depending on the application for which it is used. In the simplest neural networks there are only two layers – one 'input' layer and one 'output' layer – and are known as 'perceptrons' (Rosenblatt, 1958). These networks are only able to discriminate linear relationships between variables because they possess only one layer of weights. The more sophisticated 'multi-layer' perceptron (as popularised in Rumelhart & McClelland, 1986) adds a number of 'hidden' layers of units and therefore the two sets of weights increase the power of the network to infer non-linear relationships between variables. There is no theoretical limit to the number of layers a network can possess, although these two are among the most popular.

Learning

In most applications of this type of neural technique, the task for the network is to relate the variables it receives in the input layer to some desired behaviour at the output layer by repeatedly presenting the examples to the network in a process known as training. Somewhat analogous to learning in human infants, neural network training allows the network to determine the correct response to the input patterns that are presented to it. Once trained, the neural network should be capable of predicting an output given a previously unseen set of inputs. This training is known as *supervised learning* because the output is known for the training data points and therefore the required response can be given to the network during training. Supervised neural networks differ from traditional supervised learning, such as that used by identification trees, in that traditional supervised learning deals only or mainly with classification and supervised neural networks have a more general capability than this. Neural networks can also act as transducers (converting one form of input to another form of output). One of the most important aspects of neural network output is that it can be 'real-valued', whereas traditional classifiers can usually only output one of several discrete values that represent the class into which a sample falls. However, neural networks can also be used where the required response is not known, for instance in clustering tasks, with an unsupervised approach. These networks use training based solely on the input data, have no input, output and hidden layer distinctions, and are frequently used in domains where the required response is not known. The following sections describe the component parts of the neural network in addition to the training regimes employed in their use.

Units and weights

The unit (also known as a neuron or node) is the main processing element of the neural network. It receives a set of input signals and, combined with an internal function, converts the input signals to an output signal. The internal function can be as simple as a step function, or a more complex transformation such as the commonly used sigmoid function. Based on these functions, the activation function makes a 'decision' whether to fire and propagate the signal further up the network, based on the weight of the incoming signals. The step function ensures an 'all-or-nothing' response is given, whereas the sigmoid function produces a more graduated response. Figure 7.1 shows these two functions in mathematical and graphical form.

The task of the sigmoid function in Figure 7.1, for instance, is to take the incoming weights, check whether an internal threshold is exceeded, and if it is to calculate the output as the function of 1 divided by 1 plus the exponent of the value it has calculated. The effect is to produce an output that varies between 0 and 1, where large numbers of incoming negative values produce an output that is close to 0 and large numbers of incoming positive values produce an output that is close to 1. Another term for a sigmoid function is a 'logistic' function. Many other types of

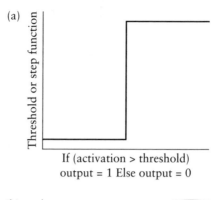

If (activation > threshold)
output = 1 Else output = 0

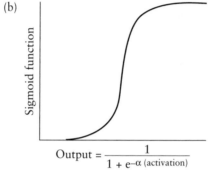

$$\text{Output} = \frac{1}{1 + e^{-\alpha \,(\text{activation})}}$$

Figure 7.1   Two possible activation functions to determine the output of a node given the sum of its input: (a) the threshold function gives a simple 1 or 0 response depending on the magnitude of the incoming signal; (b) the sigmoid function responds in a more graduated manner and the slope of the curve is dependent on the α value in the equation

function exist within neurons to convert incoming values into an output value, and such functions are called 'transfer functions', or 'activation functions', in the neural network literature.

One of the major characteristics of neural networks is that the links between nodes are themselves weighted, which is why the input to a neuron is usually called a weight. So even if a '1' is output by a transmitting neuron, if the weight attached to a link that carries that value to another neuron is 0.1, then the receiving neuron receives 0.1.

The important principle is that although the functions themselves are very simple, when a number of them are assembled together and connected with weighted connections, highly complex computation is possible. The weighted connections propagate signals from unit to unit modifying the strength of the signal according to their weight. Weights are modified in the training process and provide much of the learning capability of the network.

Architectures revisited

As described previously, the arrangement of units and weights in the neural network (often referred to as the architecture) has a profound effect on the performance of the network and even its purpose. There are a huge number of architectures that have been devised for a variety of purposes, and there are far too many to list in this book, so only the most useful architectures for bioinformaticians are described. The most commonly used of these are the feed-forward backpropagation architectures where the units are arranged in layers as described previously, and the learning algorithm is known as *supervised learning*. The feed-forward aspect of the name of this network is due to the direction of flow of the data, whereas backpropagation describes the fact that the errors incurred during learning are propagated back through the network. The directional aspects of these processes are shown in Figure 7.2, and the learning process is discussed in detail later in this section.

A very different architecture is known as the Kohonen Self Organizing Map (KSOM) (Kohonen, 1990) and belongs to the group of *unsupervised learning* algorithms. KSOMs are very different from feed-forward backpropagation networks in that all the input nodes are connected to every node in a one- or two-dimensional array of interconnected nodes.

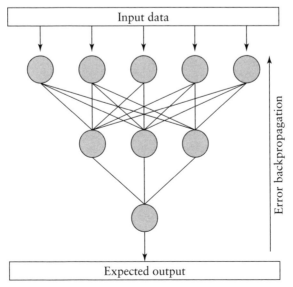

Figure 7.2   The architecture of a three-layer neural network: the direction of the data flow is shown along with that of the error which is backpropagated through the network (note that the centre layer of units have no direct contact with the input or output and are therefore named 'hidden' units)

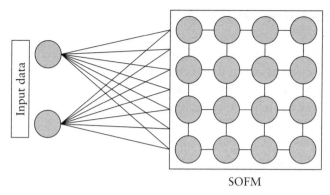

SOFM

Figure 7.3   The architecture of a self-organizing feature map: the map itself forms the output of the network and every output node is connected to every other; the input data comes from the input layer, and error correction is attempted by changing the weights of units in the map (note the differences between this approach and the one shown in Figure 7.2)

This array of nodes is known as the feature map and constitutes the output of the KSOM – there is no distinct output layer as with the feedforward backpropagation networks. This network architecture is shown in Figure 7.3.

The variety of architectures possible for neural networks can be seen in these two examples. The architecture is strongly linked to the purpose for which it has been built, for instance feed-forward networks are often used for classification and simulation, whereas KSOM networks are used for clustering and pattern recognition. Therefore the range of applications for a neural network is reflected by the range of architectures. The following section describes how these organized sets of units and weights that constitute a neural network can learn relationships from the input (and in the case of supervised learning, output) data that is presented to them.

Supervised learning

As described previously, supervised learning is the process of learning relationships between input and output data. In this type of learning, input data is passed to the input layer, propagated through the units and weights of the neural network, and the response of the network is compared to the required response, which is dictated by the output data. The discrepancy between the two is calculated and the network then makes changes to its internal weights to reduce the error the next time this input data is presented. This process is repeated for all the input data and, once completed, constitutes one 'epoch'. Most neural networks require a moderate (100–10 000+) number of epochs to effectively learn the relationships between input and output data. Supervised learning can be applied to many different types of architecture, and remains largely unchanged regardless of the number of hidden layers. However, two different algorithms are used for perceptrons and multi-layer perceptrons. The algorithm is concerned with computing the error at the output nodes and propagating this error back down the network from layer to layer. The computation of this error is different for output layers and hidden layers. The simplest learning rule is that of Rosenblatt's perception and it is this which is described below.

Perceptron learning rule

1   Initialize the network weights and unit thresholds to some small random values.

2   Present the input data $(i_1, i_2, i_3 \ldots i_n)$ and the desired output (o) data to the network

3   Calculate the output from the network using the expression:
$f(s)[\sum_{k=1}^{n} w_k(t)i_k(t)]$.

4   Adapt the weights:
   (a)   if correct $w_k(t + 1) = w_k(t)$,
   (b)   if output is 0 and should be 1 $w_k(t + 1) = w_k(t) + i_k(t)$,
   (c)   if output is 1 and should be 0 $w_k(t + 1) = w_k(t) - i_k(t)$,

where $w_k(t)$ is the weight value at time t, $w_k(t + 1)$ is the weight value at time $t + 1$ (i.e. after updating) and $f(s)$ is the function used to compute the output in the network (in this case, the step function). This learning rule ensures that the weights are changed so that the next time this same input pattern is shown, the weights alter the network behaviour so that it is closer to giving the correct response. Figure 7.4 shows the learning process. This is the simplest learning rule and a variety of modifications have been subsequently added, including the introduction of a Δ term to modify the weights more slowly giving the equation

$$w_k(t + 1) = w_k(t) + \Delta i_k(t).$$

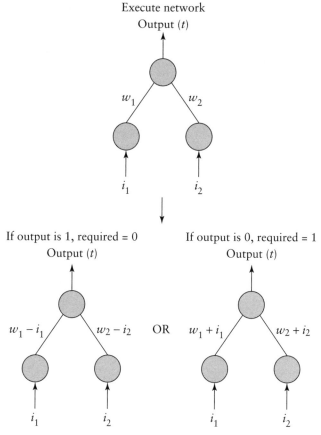

Figure 7.4   The perceptron learning rule for a single input pattern: once the network has been executed, the error between the output and the required output is calculated; depending on the result of this calculation, the weights in the network are modified to provide a better response the next time the network is presented with that input

This is sufficient to enable learning in a perceptron but, as discussed in previous sections, this is the simplest of neural networks and can only process linear interactions between variables. The following section describes the rule required for multi-layer perceptions.

Backpropagation

For larger architectures with a 'hidden layer' a more complex learning rule is required. The multi-layer perceptron often uses the sigmoid function. Therefore when the difference between the actual and desired output patterns is calculated, the weights must be changed in accordance with the derivative of this function, as opposed to the simple increment/decrement approach when considering the step function. Also, because more than one layer of weights is considered, the learning rule must take into account this fact and contain some method of backpropagating the error through the network. The multi-layer perceptron learning rule therefore implements the sigmoid derivative and backpropagation to allow it to learn.

1 Initialize the thresholds and weights.

2 Present the input data $(i_1, i_2, i_3 \ldots i_n)$ and the desired output (o) data to the network.

3 Calculate the output from the network using the expression $f[\sum_{k=1}^{n} w_k i_k]$ for each layer in the network. The output from the final layer is the vector of output values.

4 Adapt the weights, starting from the output layer and moving backwards using the equation

$$w_{ij}(t + 1) = w_{ij}(t) + \delta_{pj} o_{pj}$$

where o_{pj} is the output of node j for pattern p and δ_{pj} is defined as:

for the output layer: $\delta_{pj} = c o_{pj}(1 - o_{pj})(d_{pj} - o_{pj})$

for hidden layers: $\delta_{pj} = c o_{pj}(1 - o_{pj}) \sum_{k} \delta_{pk} - w_{jk}$,

where d is the desired output, o is the actual output and c is a constant used in the sigmoid function. The sum shown for hidden layers is over the k nodes in the layer above the current layer for which the δ_{pj} will already have been computed.

The equations above, illustrated in Figure 7.5, increment (or decrement) the weights of the network based on the error at the layer above. In the case of the output layer, the error is directly computed with the desired response, whereas the hidden layer computes its error based on the weighted error propagated back from the output layer. This process therefore allows the network to adapt its weights to correct the difference between its current output and the desired output. When applied a number of times over all the input and output data, the network reconfigures

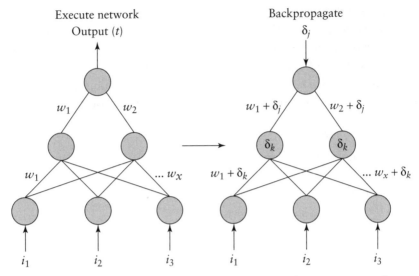

Figure 7.5 The backpropagation learning rule for a single input pattern: the network is again executed, and the error between outputs and desired output calculated

itself to be more accurate and can then be used to predict the outcome of new examples. This type of learning is only possible when the desired response is known and therefore supervised learning can take place. The desired response, however, is not known for some problems and therefore unsupervised learning rules exist to find interesting patterns in the data and to partition it into clusters and it is this which is considered in the next section.

Unsupervised learning

Kohonen self-organizing maps (KSOMs) operate in the following way. If all the output nodes (one- or two-dimensional) are interconnected and all input nodes are connected to all nodes in the output layer with no hidden layers, the task is to project the structure of the input data onto some topological structure at the output layer. The location of a neuron in the output layer should ideally reflect a particular domain or feature of the input data. Assuming that there are a number of input samples, we choose one at random and feed it into the input layer. Even if the weights connecting the input layer to the output layer have been initially randomized, one output node will have an activation value that is higher than all other output nodes. This is called the 'winning' node and the weights leading to that output node from all the input nodes are recorded.

All these weights are then updated in such a way that if the same pattern is presented again later there is even more chance of the output node having the highest activation value. To ensure that this happens, the competitive learning algorithm used by KSOMs increases the weights of not just the winning node but also, by a lesser amount, the weights of nodes neighbouring the winning node, with this increase falling away further away from the winning node. If the next input pattern shares some features with the previous pattern, there is an increased likelihood that output nodes near the winning node will be more highly active than other nodes far away, and over time input samples sharing similar features will activate neighbouring nodes in the output layer.

For example, imagine that we have two objects, a rectangle and a triangle (Figure 7.6), on a nine by eight grid. These figures are converted into a bit vector representation which's presented to the input nodes of a KSOM, with a 1 in a training pattern signifying that a particular square of the grid is occupied by a shape. These 18 eight-bit vectors are fed into an eight-node input layer which is fully connected to a four by five output layer. Ideally, after training, the output layer should reflect in its topology some aspects of the structure of the two shapes.

Unsupervised learning relies on the assumption that the data has an underlying structure that determines to which classification or pattern

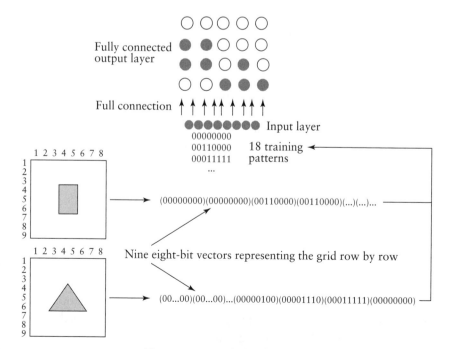

Figure 7.6 An idealized KSOM

the input data belongs. Unsupervised learning does not require a desired response (and therefore output data) to train and is concerned with discovering a common set of features across the input data in one class or pattern. The output of the Kohonen network is seen in the feature map which is a grid of interconnected units. The feature map organizes itself so that it effectively clusters the data into groups with similar features. To accomplish this, the weights from the inputs to the map are randomly initialized. When the input data closely matches the input weight, the area around that node is optimized to represent the average of the training data. By iterating through this process, the Kohonen network is able to organize itself such that different areas of the map represent different classes in the data. The Kohonen algorithm can be more formally summarized in the following steps.

1   Initialize the network by setting the weights to be small random values. Also set the initial neighbourhood size N to be large.

2   Present input patterns $I_1(t)$, $I_2(t)$, $I_3(t) \ldots I_n(t)$ where $I_x(t)$ is the input to node x at time t.

3   Calculated the distances, d_j, between the input and each node in the map j.

$$d_j = \sum_{x=1}^{n} (I_x(t) - w_{ij}(t))^2.$$

4   Select the node which has the minimum distance d_j and mark it m.

5   Update the weights for node j^* and its neighbours which are defined by the neighbourhood size. The new weights are defined as

$$w_{ij}(t+1) = w_{ij}(t) + \eta(t) * (I_x(t) - w_{ij}(t)).$$

6   Repeat 2–5.

The η term is a factor, less than one, which slows learning over time and is included so that the network makes smaller decisions with each training epoch. A further factor in these equations is that the neighbourhood size is made smaller throughout training which leads to more refined moves in the latter stages of the learning process.

Unsupervised learning is especially useful where data has been collected from an experiment, but no output classification has been determined. As such, this is one of the techniques in this book that can discover patterns and classify data without using some form of explicit notion of how closely it matches a desired response. This is especially important in bioinformatics since various problems in the analysis of microarray data or of protein structure prediction do not have definitive classical examples on which the network can be trained.

These two learning rules show the wide variety of learning behaviour that can be performed using neural network methods. They represent only two of a number of learning methods and functions which can be employed depending on the type of problem that is being solved. One of the strengths of the neural approach is the sheer flexibility in the number of options available for architecture, activation function and training regime. A drawback of this flexibility is that there is no generally accepted method for choosing a specific architecture or activation function given a problem definition. Indeed, selecting the neural network parameters has often been described as an art rather than a science. To aid this selection, the following section gives some guidelines as to the application of neural networks to problems in bioinformatics.

7.2 Application guidelines

Neural networks have been used for a huge variety of applications in a large number of scientific and engineering domains and they can be considered one of the standard artificial intelligence (AI) techniques for a variety of purposes. Whilst there are undoubtedly a number of situations in which the application of a neural network is the recommended course of action, there are also some caveats to their usage for particular problems. Put simply, a neural network that is properly trained on a suitable problem can provide very good or even genuinely surprising results on new data. It is the ability of the neural network to generalize beyond the data that it has been trained on which makes it so powerful. However, they have some drawbacks.

1   Neural networks can overfit (a term for overtraining). If a neural network is trained for too long, it can begin to fit the weights to the noise in the training data as well as the underlying structure which is present. When this happens, the error on the training data will continue to decrease, but the error on the test data will actually increase.

Commercial neural network packages now include a cross-validation facility to combat this effect. This method trains the network for one epoch, freezes the weights, tests the trained network on a separate test set and restarts the training. This approach is repeated for each epoch of training. The error on the cross-validation set can then be used to stop the training of the neural network when it begins to increase. This mitigates many of the problems of overtraining, and gives a good idea of the error that can be expected on test data.

2   The architecture requires some input from the user. Deciding on the appropriate architecture for a neural network should largely be informed by the type of data and complexity of the problem being solved. However, there are no hard and fast rules as to the number of hidden layers, or units in those layers for example that are required for a particular problem. For prediction accuracy and ease of result interpretation, a supervised learning algorithm (i.e. multi-layer perceptron) should be selected if the desired response is known. The minimum number of hidden layers should be used that can achieve the required accuracy. For each addition of a hidden layer, the power of the network is increased, but with an attendant increase in the likelihood of overfitting and, of course, computation time. A good rule of thumb is that any hidden layers used should have fewer units than the input layer. In fact, many applications use a stepped approach where the number of units in the hidden layer decreases from input to output. If, using unsupervised learning, the number of nodes in the feature map will influence the number of clusters that are discovered in the data, this parameter should also be selected with care. These are very general guidelines and a good number of applications will require deviation from them, but they can be used as initial parameter settings when a new problem is considered.

3   Finally, it can be difficult to determine the reasoning for the decision making behaviour of the neural network. A trained neural network contains many weights, biases and thresholds, often in high-dimensional matrices, and it is a non-trivial process to determine the exact reasoning behind its behaviour on a certain dataset. Certainly, if one or more hidden layers is used, determining the combined effect of each input at each hidden layer and onto the output layer is very difficult indeed. In this case, sensitivity analysis (manipulating the inputs in a structured way and observing the output response) can provide some information that may be very difficult to derive from the weight

matrices. If neural networks are to be applied to a problem, the problem should generally not require that the decision making behaviour of the network can be explained in human-understandable terms.

Implementation

Whilst the above set of problems, architecture choices and mathematical equations can seem quite daunting, there is a large body of research and software available to aid the application of neural networks to problems in bioinformatics. For instance there is a vast array of neural network software implementations available on the internet. One of the most famous and respected free implementations is the Stuttgart Neural Network Simulator or SNNS[1] which is available from the University of Tubingen, Germany; it has a wealth of architecture options and has versions for a variety of operating systems. Commercial neural network products abound, but a useful interactive point-and-click style software package is Neurosolutions[2] from Neurodimension. This package has a large library of built-in network architectures and the user interface is such that creating new architectures is simply accomplished by manipulating the components of the network on screen. It also has a data-driven Neural Wizard which guides the user through the process of creating a neural network for a particular problem.

In addition to these there are various neural network implementations in all programming languages on the internet and a good selection of information sources to help with neural networks[3].

7.3 Bioinformatics applications

Introduction

Neural networks have received a significant amount of attention as an AI algorithm for bioinformatics. As with many of the algorithms in this book, each method is chosen for its suitability to a particular problem. It comes as no surprise then that most bioinformatics applications focus on the ability of the neural network to cluster and recognize patterns within

---

[1] More information available from http://www-ra.informatik.uni-tuebingen.de/SNNS/.
[2] More information available from http://www.nd.com.
[3] A search on the web for 'Neural Network FAQ' will give a variety of pages pointing to the valuable neural network reference.

biological data. The following examples have been selected as they give an overview of what is possible by using both the above techniques in bioinformatics problems.

Classification and dimensionality reduction of gene expression data

Introduction

Gene expression data is currently one of the hottest topics in bioinformatics and it looks set to be one of the most revealing analysis techniques used in biology. Microarray data is notoriously difficult to process, even after a successful experiment it is noisy and requires many statistical transformations to yield correct and normalized gene expression values. However, even once this is achieved, there are further difficulties in analysing this type of data, namely that the number of genes is so large that typical analysis methods can be completely ineffective in the face of the 'curse of dimensionality'. Gene expression experiments are often used to attempt to distinguish between diseased and normal individuals, or to distinguish between two types of a disease by solely using the expression values of genes taken from those individuals. This is of primary importance to medical science as a number of different cancers are very difficult to diagnose. Narayanan *et al.* (2004) and earlier, Khan *et al.* (2001) have both shown that single layer neural networks (or perceptrons) can be used as an effective method for reducing the number of genes to be considered in an analysis.

Method and results

In Narayanan *et al.* (2004) a standard perceptron was iteratively applied to a gene expression dataset and genes stripped from the dataset based on the weight values taken from the neural network. Essentially, the perceptron was used as a method for determining the importance of each gene to the classes in the dataset. In this paper, a multiple myeloma dataset was used where the task was to distinguish the 74 multiple myeloma sufferers from the 31 normal individuals, based solely on their gene expression profiles. The data consisted initially of 7129 genes, had a classification of either myelomic or non-myleomic and was separated into three separate sets, used for training, tuning and testing respectively. These sets were used in a three-fold cross-validation procedure where each set was used in turn to train, tune and test the neural network. This type of testing is common in classification tasks such as this one and ensures that the results are generalizable.

The method consists of a number of steps.

1 *Pre-process the data* – gene expression data is often in a format whereby genes are listed as rows and samples as columns. This facilitates the viewing process, but the neural network requires the data in the transposed format, so a transposition must be carried out. In addition to this, the data can often have missing values, again the neural network will require values in each column and row, so these values are often imputed.

2 *Training and testing* – this approach uses a three fold cross-validation technique where the data is split into three datasets. The neural network is trained, tuned and tested on each of these three datasets in turn, and the results averaged over the three runs. This ensures that the accuracy of the approach is robust over a number of different datasets.

3 *Gene pruning* – once the perceptron has been trained, the weights of the network are inspected to determine which genes are most highly related to the classification. Those genes which do not meet the threshold requirements (usually a number of standard deviations away from the mean) are pruned and the process is repeated.

For each iteration of training, a perceptron was created with N input units, where N is the number of genes being trained (therefore, in the first instance, this is 7129), and one output unit (to give the classification 1 and 0). The network is trained for 10 000 epochs and then the weights analysed to determine those individual genes which have not contributed to the 0 and 1 classification. Those genes which are within two standard deviations of the mean weight value are considered to be non-contributory and are removed for the next iteration. Once this had been completed, 481 genes remained and the process was repeated. After one further iteration, 39 genes remained and were ranked by weight value. In each of the iterations of the above process, the perceptron achieved 100 per cent accuracy on the test set and therefore by progressively selecting smaller subsets of genes, a good deal of extraneous information in the database was removed. The final 39 genes were then investigated to determine their biological significance. This was performed by using the NCBI database of gene structure and function[4] and some of the genes were found to have been previously linked with other cancers, or myeloma itself.

Khan *et al.* (2001) takes a slightly different approach to a similar problem. The data to which they applied neural networks were gene expression values of small, round blue cell tumours, so called because of their appearance in histology. The difficulty was that four separate diseases, neuroblastoma, rhabdomyosarcoma, non-Hodgkin lymphoma and the Ewing family of tumours can all give rise to this similar histology. However, accurate diagnosis is essential as each of the four types responds differently to treatment. Khan *et al.* used the gene expression data of 6567 genes from 63 samples, but this was reduced by removing those genes with a small variation about the mean. It is considered that genes such as this which do not vary significantly either over time or samples, will be of little use in classification. In addition to this, principal component analysis was used to reduce the number of inputs still further. A three-fold cross-validation process was then conducted which when combined with 1250 separate runs for each fold yielded a total of 3750 neural networks. The networks were tested as a committee on classification and diagnostic problems and found to be highly accurate. In addition to this, the sensitivity of the neural network to inputs was determined, and the number of genes further reduced by pruning those that the network was not using to classify the data. Several experiments showed that the optimum number of genes was 96 as this was the smallest number of genes which gave 100 per cent accuracy. After further investigation, it was found that 61 of these genes (some were eliminated as copies) were related to the classification, of which 41 had not previously been identified as related to these diseases.

Conclusion

The above approaches show the value of using simple neural techniques to discover interactions between variables (in this case gene expression values) and a classification. The difference between this and other classification approaches is that the final accuracy of the set of genes is only one consideration. The neural network approach provides a set of genes to be investigated as the possible cause for a particular disease. This is in contrast to the performance on this problem of other techniques such as decision trees which discover a very small number of genes which are

[4] For more information go to: http://www.ncbi.nlm.nih.gov/Database/.

often accurate on the training data, but have disappointing accuracy on test data. The notion is that the number of genes is reduced to the point that it can be fruitfully analysed (in combination with the weights which help to indicate the importance of a gene in the classification) but not oversimplified so that something is missed. This application of a perceptron in both these studies clearly shows that even the simplest of the neural network technologies can be used to good effect in bioinformatics problems.

Identifying protein subcellular location

Introduction

Protein function is often closely related to its location within the cell and work undertaken by Cai, Liu and Chou (2002) used a Kohonen neural network (as described above in the Unsupervised Learning section) to predict where a protein was located, based on its amino acid make-up. As the number of discovered proteins increases, determining the subcellular location of such a protein can provide important clues as to its structure and function in the cell. The study was short, but it neatly showed the effectiveness of the Kohonen network in tasks such as this.

Method and results

The authors clearly identified a set of data from Chou and Elrod (1999) where each of the 2139 proteins was assigned an unambiguous class from this set: (1) chloroplast, (2) cytoplasm, (3) cytoskeleton, (4) endoplasmic reticulum, (5) extracellular, (6) Golgi apparatus, (7) lysosome, (8) mitochondria, (9) nucleus, (10) peroxisome, (11) plasma membrane and (12) vacuole. The proteins themselves were represented by 20 variables which each represented an amino acid in the makeup of the protein. A Kohonen network was trained on the dataset and then tested by inputting the test data and observing which nodes in the feature map was most highly activated by the test example. Each study was performed with a self-consistency test (effectively executing the network on the data on which it was trained), and more significantly, a leave-one-out cross-validation approach was also used. Using this method the network achieved an accuracy of almost 80 per cent on the leave-one-out cross-validation tests. Whilst this is some 2 per cent less than the state-of-the-art (the covariant discriminant algorithm in this case), the authors claimed that this approach was more accurate than other widely-used systems such as ProtLock. Encouragingly, the approach also achieved similar accuracy on three independent test datasets which corroborated the leave-one-out cross-validation findings.

Conclusion

The above example indicates that given a good problem definition, a neural network approach can be developed to solve a difficult problem in bioinformatics. The network clearly grasped the relationship between the amino acid make-up of the protein and its location in the cell. This is significant because if location can be determined from amino acid make-up, then an educated guess at function can then be made. Whilst the results were not optimal when the current best algorithms are considered, it must be remembered that the Kohonen approach is unsupervised and therefore must make the class decisions itself rather than being taught them explicitly. Finally, this research illustrates good use of the cross-validation procedure (which in this case is of the leave-one-out variety), as the results on independent test sets were very close to those predicted in cross-validation.

7.4 Background

Perceptrons, the simplest neural networks, were pioneered by Frank Rosenblatt (1958) in the late fifties but Minsky and Papert (1969) published *Perceptrons* a book which highlighted the shortcomings of the perceptron and, crucially, the fact that it could not recreate the XOR function with just two layers. This deficiency led neural networks to be practically discarded in favour of symbolic computation techniques for over 20 years before the seminal publication of *Parallel Distributed Processing* (Rumelhart and McClelland) in 1986 which built on the concept that a multi-layer perceptron could learn the XOR and a massive variety of other functions. This discovery revitalized the field and, combined with a general sense of disappointment in the achievements of symbolic computation, led to a large number of researchers entering the field of neural computation. Since then, neural networks have been applied to countless problems and are especially successful in the areas of financial forecasting and computer vision to name just two.

7.5 Summary of chapter

1 Neural networks are a mathematical technique, broadly based on the functioning of the brain, which can be trained by two methods – supervised and unsupervised learning.

2 Supervised learning is often used in instances where the required output is known, unsupervised learning is used when this is not possible or desirable.

3 Once trained, a neural network can be shown new examples of data and can make predictions based on what it has learnt from the training data.

4 Neural networks have found application in bioinformatics problems, from gene expression analysis through to protein location prediction.

7.6 References

Cai, Y-D., Liu, X-J., Chou, K-C. (2002) Artificial neural network model for predicting protein subcellular location. *Computers and Chemistry*, **26**, 179–182.

Chou, K.C. and Elrod, D.W. (1999) Protein subcellular location prediction. *Protein Eng.*, **12**, 107–118.

Khan, J., Wei, J.S., Ringner, M. *et al.* (2001) Classification and diagnostic prediction of cancers using gene expression profiling and artificial neural networks. *Nature Medicine*, **7**, 673–679.

Kohonen, T. (1990) The self-organizing map. *Proceedings of the IEEE*, **78**, 1464–1480.

Minsky, M. and Papert, S. (1969) *Perceptrons; An Introduction to Computational Geometry*. MIT Press, Cambridge, MA.

Narayanan, A., Keedwell, E., Tatineni, S.S. *et al.* (2004) Single-layer artificial neural networks for gene expression analysis. *Neurocomputing*, **61**, 217–240.

Rosenblatt, F. (1958) The perception: a probabilistic model for information storage and organization in the brain. *Psychological Review*, **65**, 386–408.

Rumelhart, D.E. and McClelland, J.L. (1986) *Parallel Distributed Processing: Volume 1 Foundations*. The Massachusetts Institute of Technology.

8

Genetic Algorithms

8.1 Single-objective genetic algorithms – method

'Genetic algorithms', 'evolutionary computation' and many of the terms described in this chapter have distinct biological overtones. It is worth stating at the outset that the genetic algorithm (GA) is a search and optimization tool which can be used to solve bioinformatics problems, not a metaphor for how genetic operations are carried out in the real world. The GA is in fact inspired by the mechanisms of evolution and these have proved useful in a variety of search and optimization domains. Genetic algorithms use principles of evolution such as *reproduction*, *selection*, *crossover* and *mutation* (collectively known as genetic operators) to discover better solutions to a problem given a random starting set of solutions. Each of these operators acts on one or more *chromosomes* (solutions) in the *population* (a set of solutions) to yield a set of new solutions which is known as the next *generation*. The algorithm is iterative, and therefore these operators act upon the population many times, moving the algorithm from one *generation* to the next.

Genetic algorithms are now widely applied in engineering and scientific disciplines. Generally, this is due to the fact that they can be readily adapted to new problems, they are efficient with respect to other search algorithms, and also they are less prone to descending into local minima/maxima. A problem with many standard search algorithms, such as hill-climbing (Chapter 3), is that they often find solutions in the search space which are locally – but not globally – optimum when the space is not smooth (i.e. in most real-world problems). Genetic algorithms, due to their stochastic and population-based nature, are able to avoid this behaviour for the most part. They have therefore found favour in a large number of domains where traditional techniques would require too much computation to produce an optimal solution and where a near-optimal one will suffice.

Chromosome

A good deal of the success of the GA is based on its flexibility. The problem- independent nature of the GA is the reason it can be applied to so many domains without alteration of the algorithm itself. This problem independence is established through the use of a *chromosome* and *objective function*. The chromosome is a genetic representation of a single solution to the problem and its performance at solving that problem is evaluated by a function which relates the chromosome variables to the problem at hand. Figure 8.1 shows a chromosome representation of a problem.

To evaluate the chromosome, the objective function takes the chromosome (which is usually represented in some numerical or binary format), decodes it according to a problem specific decoding scheme and then computes the fitness of the solution which is then passed back to the algorithm. The most important skill in applying a GA to a problem is to be able to correctly map the problem to a set of integers or binary variables and accurately compute a fitness so that it reflects the problem at hand. Later in this chapter various methods for accomplishing this for bioinformatics problems will be discussed.

Operators

Once a random population of solutions has been created, the genetic operators that act on the population of solutions must drive the population

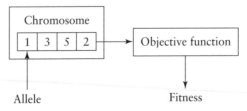

Figure 8.1 Relationship between the chromosome, objective function and fitness

to find new, more optimal solutions. The most important of these are the selection, mutation and crossover procedures that determine which individuals survive to the next generation. In the GA, a number of individuals (normally two at a time) are selected from the current population, their genetic material is then combined together to form a number (again, normally two) of new individuals in a process known as crossover. A random mutation can also take place to alter the genetic make-up of these individuals. This process is repeated until the next generation is full, whereupon each individual is evaluated by the objective function and the process is repeated. The following sections describe some of the most popular operators used in GA applications.

Selection

As with other search algorithms, the GA needs to remember good solutions and discard bad ones if it is to make progress towards the optimum. A very simple selector would be to select the top N chromosomes from each population for progression to the next population. This would work up to a point, but any solutions which have very high fitness will always make it through to the next population. This concept is known as *elitism* and will be covered later in this chapter. However, to make sure that the GA doesn't *converge* on a set of solutions too quickly, a random element is usually introduced into the selection procedure. The following section describes the *roulette wheel selector*, which is one of the most popular procedures along with the *tournament selector*.

Roulette wheel selector

This selector works by adding all the fitness values of chromosomes in the population together to create a 'virtual roulette wheel'. This wheel is then spun to see which of the individuals is chosen for selection into the next generation. As can be seen by Figure 8.2, if the wheel is 'spun' there is a much greater chance of solution with higher fitness being selected over the other solutions in the 'roulette wheel'. This affords filter solutions a better chance of being kept in the next generation than the others. However, an important point is that there is still a chance that any of the solutions can be selected, as the selection procedure depends on a random number. This method allows the selection to be biased towards

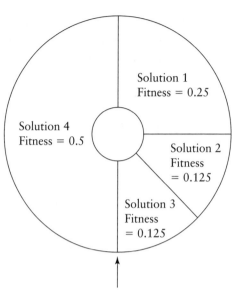

Figure 8.2 Roulette wheel selection: the total fitness of a population of chromosomes can be represented as a wheel, where the fitness of an individual chromosome is represented an appropriate 'slice' of the wheel; the higher the fitness value, the larger the portion of wheel occupied by that chromosome

those solutions that solve the problem well, but the stochastic element of selection ensures that diversity in the population is maintained.

Tournament selection

Tournament selection has a similar mix of randomness but contains a bias towards fitter individuals. In tournament selection, a number of chromosomes (normally 2) are selected from the population and their fitness compared. Quite simply, the chromosome with greatest fitness is selected for entry to the next generation. The random selection of individuals to participate in the tournament means that two poorly performing solutions could be selected at once. In this situation, even though the solutions are poor with respect to the rest of the population, the best individual of the two will be selected. It is in this way that solutions with low fitness can still be selected by the tournament selector. This selection process ensures that, over the course of a number of generations, fit individuals are more likely to be selected for entry to the next generation and this therefore preserves information discovered in previous generations. Once selected, solutions undergo crossover and mutation, which are described in the next section.

Cross over

The cross over operator is designed so that two 'parent' solutions can combine information to produce two new 'offspring' solutions that are different, but related to the original solutions. Again, there are a number of methods of achieving this and two of the most common are described here, single point and uniform crossover.

Single point crossover

Single point crossover is the simplest crossover and takes two chromosomes, chooses a single random point on each chromosome and cuts the two chromosomes at this point. The two parts of the chromosome are then recombined to form two new individuals which share some of the information of the parents, but are separate solutions in their own right. Figure 8.3 illustrates this process.

Uniform crossover

Difficulties can arise when using single point crossover, since genes towards the centre of the chromosome are perturbed more often than those at the edges of the chromosome. To overcome this, uniform crossover takes multiple random points on each chromosome and creates a 'mask' through which the chromosomes pass. Figure 8.4 shows the execution of

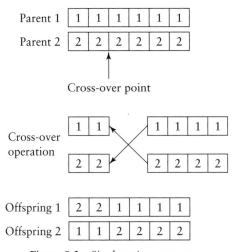

Figure 8.3 Single point cross-over

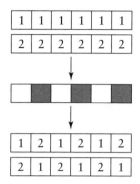

Figure 8.4   Uniform cross-over

uniform crossover where two chromosomes pass through a filter, where the grey squares indicate that a 'swap' of alleles takes place and the white squares indicate that the values pass through untouched. Uniform crossover ensures that each gene on the chromosome has an equal chance of being crossed over and represents a crossover without positional bias.

Crossover operators therefore ensure that material taken from two selected parents is merged in such a way that the information that contributed to the parents fitness will be kept in the offspring. The crossover operator is stochastic as the crossover point is selected at random. One possible difficulty is that, for certain types of problem, crossover may result in a chromosome that is not permitted for the task at hand. For instance, if some allelic values towards the end of a chromosome depend on allelic values earlier in the chromosome (such as, for instance, a route finding problem where only one occurrence of a city or node in a map can occur in a chromosome), crossover will need to be supplemented by some check procedure that ensures that the results of crossover still make sense. Some post crossover procedure may be required to mend the results of crossover so that solutions still fall in the space of acceptable solutions. Once selection and crossover have taken place, the solutions are mutated.

Mutation

Selection and crossover ensure that the best individuals have the greatest chance of progressing into the next population and can share their information to give the best possible solutions. Both processes include an element of random behaviour but a further random element is required to complete the GA, known as mutation. Without the mutation operator, the GA is only capable of manipulating the genetic material that was present in the initial population. Mutators generally are not as complicated as crossover and mutation; they tend to just choose a random point on the chromosome and perturb this allele either completely randomly or by some given amount. For instance, one possible mutation operation is to take a chromosome, such as the second offspring in Figure 8.3, and randomly 'mutate' one allele by adding a value in the range 1 to 3. If the second allele of Offspring 2 is chosen at random for mutation, it may change from 1 to 4, resulting in a chromosome consisting of allele values '1 4 2 2 2 2'. Mutation needs to be coupled with some check that the final mutated value is not out of bounds for a particular allele. For instance, if the possible range of values for allele 2 is only 1 to 3, the value 4 for this allele cannot be allowed.

Generational vs. steady state

The final element of the GA is how the algorithm progresses from one generation to the next. There are two ways of achieving this: a generational method, where a new population is generated at every iteration, and a steady-state method where the population stays largely the same but new solutions are added to it. Figure 8.5 shows a generational genetic algorithm, where a new population is created every generation.

The steady-state genetic algorithm shown in Figure 8.6 selects a number of individuals from the population, applies the reproduction, crossover and mutation operators to them and then reinserts them into the population using a variety of criteria. These replacement criteria usually take the form of replacing the weaker (or weakest) solutions in the population and therefore increasing the fitness of the population in this way.

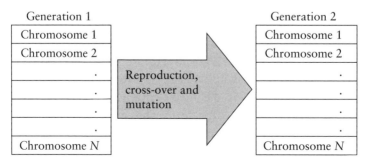

Figure 8.5   Generational genetic algorithm

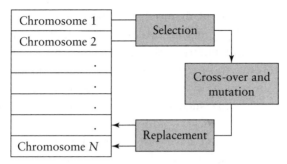

Figure 8.6   Steady-state genetic algorithm

By using these simple biologically inspired operators, a well-conceived representation of the problem and an accurate objective function, the GA can solve a vast array of search and optimization problems, quickly and efficiently.

8.2 Single-objective genetic algorithms – example

Introduction

The best way to understand the GA is to begin with a simple example of its execution. The following section describes a very simple example of a GA problem. Given the function, $f(x) = x^2$, we want to get the GA to maximize the function where x will be the sum of four decision variables which will range from -10 to $+10$. That is, the task is to discover what the four values making up x must be for the function to return its maximum positive value, given that x is squared. This problem has two global optima (one where each decision variable is -10 and one where each is $+10$). This simple problem is representative of many search and optimization problems where there exists more than one answer to the problem and demonstrates the capability of the algorithm to discover global optima. A non-genetic algorithm approach to this problem could consist of enumerating all possible values for the four decision variables, summing them and squaring the answer in turn, and storing the result. At the end of this enumeration (or during the enumeration for added efficiency), that combination of four values that allows the function to return the maximum value is discovered. Since there are 20 possible values for each variable (ranging from -10 to $+10$), the full enumeration will need to examine 20^4 different combinations of values. A GA may be able to identify the solution more efficiently than this, even for this simple task.

Execution

Using a random number generator, a set of 10 individuals (chromosomes) is created, each with four decision variables (DVs) ranging from -10 to $+10$. These decision variables are summed and then squared (as specified by the function) to give a fitness value as follows.

	DV1	DV2	DV3	DV4	Sum	Fitness
Chrom 1	−6	−6	−8	−1	−21	441
Chrom 2	−4	1	6	−10	−7	49
Chrom 3	2	−10	1	2	−5	25
Chrom 4	−10	−4	−3	−7	−24	576
Chrom 5	0	−7	5	8	6	36
Chrom 6	−2	3	8	−9	0	0
Chrom 7	6	2	4	3	15	225
Chrom 8	−2	−1	−9	5	−7	49
Chrom 9	4	−7	7	−5	−1	1
Chrom 10	1	−4	−7	−9	−19	361
					Average	176.3

If by chance chromosomes 4 and 10 were selected and crossed over at point 2, the resulting children would be created

Child 1	−10	−4	−7	−9	−30	900

and

Child 2	1	−4	−3	−7	−13	169

A mutation can then occur changing the variable 1 in child 2 to a 3 which gives:

Child 2	3	−4	−3	−7	−11	121

By using a 'weakest' replacement strategy, Chromosome 6 is replaced by Child 1 and Chromosome 9 replaced by Child 2. The population now looks like this.

	Allele1	Allele2	Allele3	Allele4	Sum	Fitness
Chrom 1	−6	−6	−8	−1	−21	441
Chrom 2	−4	1	6	−10	−7	49
Chrom 3	2	−10	1	2	−5	25
Chrom 4	−10	−4	−3	−7	−24	576
Chrom 5	0	−7	5	8	6	36
Child 1	−10	−4	−7	−9	−30	900
Chrom 7	6	2	4	3	15	225
Chrom 8	−2	−1	−9	5	−7	49
Child 2	3	−4	−3	−7	−11	121
Chrom 10	1	−4	−7	−9	−19	361
					Average	278.3

By using just one generation of the GA, the average fitness of the population has risen from 176 to 278. In addition to this, an individual with a fitness of 900 has been created, by far the highest from the two populations and also much higher than that of its parents. This example illustrates two key concepts of the GA.

1   By using just the genetic operators we have discovered a new best solution (of fitness 900) and improved the overall fitness of the population by replacing poorly performing solutions.

2   Not every move is good. By mutating Child 2's first allele from 1 to 3, we have actually decreased the fitness of that chromosome. This happens frequently in genetic algorithms and appears to be counterintuitive, but the increased value of 3 might be of benefit if that chromosome is crossed-over in a later generation. The mutation is only counter-productive because of the make-up of the remainder of the chromosome. In itself the move from 1 to 3 for a single gene represents an improvement as it is closer to the +10 extremity. The operators are designed to increase the likelihood of fit individuals going into the next generation, not guarantee it.

After several further generations, the GA will be able to converge on a set of very good solutions to this task. While this task may appear trivial, that is because the function is simple. If the function being maximized consisted of several dozen variables ranging from −1000 to +1000, and if more than a simple summing and squaring of the variable values is required, a full enumeration will not be possible and the GA approach will be more attractive.

8.3 Multi-objective genetic algorithms – method

Introduction

The single-objective GA is immensely useful when a single, near-optimal solution to a problem is needed. However, many science and engineering applications consist of objectives where there are conflicts. For instance, when designing a structure such as an aircraft, there are the conflicting objectives of strength and weight, where extra bracing in the structure allows it to be stronger but heavier and therefore less efficient. Genetic algorithms, with some modifications, can be used to optimize problems with more than one objective, creating a multi-objective GA. Whilst such applications in bioinformatics are currently limited, multi-objective algorithms are likely to become widely used in the discipline in the near future due to the need to balance conflicting requirements, such as protein function with protein folding.

The main similarities between single and multi-objective GAs are that they still use a population of individuals and crossover, mutation and selection operators, although some of these can be a little different in multi-objective algorithms. The main difference is the way that the performance of each individual is determined. In the single objective case, fitness is the only criterion by which solutions are compared. In multi-objective algorithms, this is replaced by the notion of dominance. Since each individual solution is evaluated on a number of objectives (for instance, weight and strength for a particular aircraft design), there is no theoretical limit to the number of objectives used. To compare individual solutions, a new measure known as dominance is used to rate each solution.

Dominance

One solution is said to *dominate* another if it is as good or better than that solution in all objectives (this concept is known as strong dominance in the literature). The following example shows how dominance works.

If three designs exist for an aircraft, we want to discover the design with maximum strength and minimum weight. Given the following three solutions, the choice is difficult to make.

Solution	Weight	Strength
1	45	2.2
2	30	1.5
3	25	1.0

A decrease in weight is accompanied by a decrease in strength and therefore each of these solutions does not dominate any other. However, if a fourth solution is included which has a weight of 22 and a strength of 2.5, this solution dominates each of the first three solutions. This fourth solution dominates the other three because it is at least as good in every dimension as the other solutions and better in at least one this is shown in Figure 8.7. A solution is said to be *non-dominated* when no other solution in the current set dominates it. This principle of dominance of solutions distinguishes multi-objective algorithms from single-objective algorithms.

The principle of dominance can be extended to any number of objectives and gives a clear indication as to which solutions are better in the search space. The principle is then used to rank the set of solutions according to the number of times they are dominated by other solutions in the population. This ranking differentiates between the solutions in the population and allows modified selection operators to work. Figure 8.8 shows an extended example of the aircraft design problem where the ranking procedure can be seen more easily. The rank of a solution is computed as the number of solutions in the population which dominate that solution. The best solution in the example has a rank of zero, which

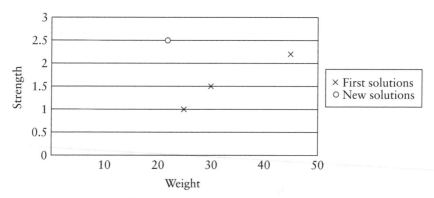

Figure 8.7 Aircraft design example

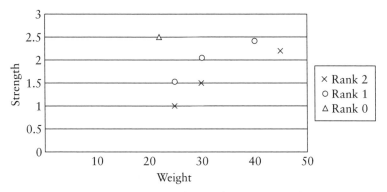

Figure 8.8 Extended aircraft design example

means that in the current population, it is the best (least-dominated) solution. There is often more than one solution with rank zero and this is known as the Pareto-front or Pareto-surface which represents the best solutions from an optimization run.

Multi-objective GAs perform operations on the population by using the rank of the individuals rather than the fitness. This approach means that, as the optimization progresses, the Pareto-front moves towards the optimum trade-off between the variables. This is seen in Figure 8.8 – the algorithm will attempt to move the points towards the top-left hand corner where maximum strength and minimum weight lie. Aside from optimality, the multi-objective algorithm tries to find a number of evenly-spaced solutions on the pareto-front. This is to provide the maximum amount of choice in the selection of a solution for its final purpose. Solutions that are tightly clustered together, and differ only marginally in their objective values, do not represent a good basis for solution selection. To summarize, the multi-objective GA, by means of simulated evolution, aims to find a pareto-set of well-spaced solutions that offer the optimal trade-off between two or more variables. This approach has been found to be very successful in many scientific, engineering and financial circles where the decision-making process has more than one consequence for a given set of actions.

8.4 Application guidelines

Introduction

Genetic algorithms have much to offer bioinformatics as they are currently one of the most efficient ways to search large problem spaces. They are regularly applied to problems which have thousands of decision variables and huge combinatorial search spaces in science and engineering. However, the most important attribute of the GA is its flexibility. By encoding the variables of the problem as bit strings or integers and using only an objective function, the GA can be applied to a number of problems in bioinformatics. Whilst they are immensely flexible, there are a number of conditions which should be met before applying the algorithm to a problem.

1 The problem should be large. If the problem can be solved with a traditional hill-climbing or local search algorithm or even a full enumeration in realistic time, then a GA may not be the most efficient method due to its stochastic nature.

2 An objective function should be constructed which relates the decision variables of the problem and assigns a 'fitness' to the solution that determines how good that solution is. Ideally this function will be as monotonic as possible (i.e. it will vary consistently with decision variable values), functions which vary wildly with respect to the decision variables are very difficult to optimize by using a GA.

3 The number and severity of constraints on the solutions should be small. A number of problems require that only a small number of the possible solutions can be considered as feasible. When this occurs, there are methods to implement constraints in genetic algorithms, but on the whole, soft constraints which penalize the fitness of solutions if they are outside the required bounds are generally preferable. If there are soft constraints on a number of variables in the fitness function, then a multi-objective approach should be considered as an alternative.

Representation

The problem being solved must be converted to a format that can be optimized with the GA. The 'representation' to the GA is very important as can determine how well the algorithm performs on the problem. Genetic algorithms can use a variety of gene types (integers, real values and bit strings) that represent variables in the problem. The most traditional approach is to use a set of bit strings to represent decision variables in the problem, since they are known to perform well with standard crossover and mutation operators. Other gene types require special crossover and mutation operators, but they can be used as effective easier-to-use representations. The issue here is between 'genotype' and 'phenotype' of chromosomes. The closer the representation of a chromosome is to the problem, the easier the chromosome is to interpret. That is, the genotype is the phenotype in the case of the simple single-objective function described earlier, where the alleles contained the actual integer values between -10 and $+10$. However, if these values were represented as bits (so, for example, seven is represented in a 10-bit allele as '0000000111', some mapping must be made between the chromosomes genotype (bit representations in the chromosome) and gene phenotype (its actual interpretation). Bit representation allows for more flexible mutation and crossover. A chromosome containing four alleles of 10 bits each has 40 mutation and 39 crossover positions as opposed to only four mutation and three crossover positions if integer representation is used. In other words, complex genotype representations will require more interpretation with regard to what they actually mean (their phenotype) in the domain, but crossover will be more effective on representations of this type.

Algorithm selection

Choices to be made with regard to genetic algorithms are largely down to the parameter settings and selection of operators, as described in previous sections. The user also needs to determine whether a steady-state or generational approach is taken. The steady-state approach is faster, as fewer objective function evaluations have to be completed per iteration, but the results may not be as good as a generational run.

Multi-objective genetic algorithms can be separated into two distinct types, the elitist and non-elitist algorithms. Elitism ensures that the very best solutions in one generation progress to the next, a concept which does not normally occur as the selection procedure can choose to select any solution from the population. Elitism is useful for multi-objective problems as it helps to preserve the Pareto-front during the optimization. Elitist genetic algorithms such as the Nondominated Sorting Genetic Algorithm 2 (NSGA-II) (Deb *et al.*, 2000) are currently the state-of-the-art and to a certain extent has superseded the original Multi-objective Genetic Algorithm (MOGA) developed by Fonseca and Fleming (1995).

Implementation

While implementing a GA in a programming language is a good way to learn the intricacies of the algorithm, there are a number of sources for libraries and applications that allow easy access to GA technology. Genetic algorithms are increasing in popularity and there are a vast number of implementations of GA software on the Internet in almost every modern programming language. The variety, quality and number of features vary greatly, so selecting the correct one for the needs of the problem can be crucial. Often, a good free or shareware implementation can be as effective as an expensive commercial product. GALib[1] from MIT in the USA is a particularly good example of a C++ version of a freeware GA library. Off-the-shelf products such as 'Evolver' from Palisade[2] also allow GA techniques to be used in the user-friendly environment of Microsoft Excel. Therefore there are a number of software options for individuals wishing to apply GAs to bioinformatics problems.

8.5 Genetic algorithms – bioinformatics applications

Introduction

With bioinformatics being a relatively new science and genetic algorithms only finding popularity relatively recently, the number of applications of GAs to bioinformatics currently remains relatively small. A large portion of the work has concentrated on using GAs to process microarray data. Specifically, they have been used to 'reverse engineer' regulatory networks and also, in conjunction with neural networks, as a method of data mining gene expression data. The following sections describe the most current research into these topics.

Reverse engineering of regulatory networks

Introduction

Gene regulatory networks are described in detail in Chapter 2, but the following sections show why GAs may be required for this particular problem. Gene expression or microarray data allows biologists unprecedented access to the workings of genes within a cell, and the expression values of many thousands of genes can be recorded simultaneously for

---

[1] More information can be found at http://lancet.mit.edu/ga/.
[2] More information can be found at http://www.palisade.com.

a particular sample. This process can be applied repeatedly for a sample placed under stimuli, which then yields a trace of genetic activity for a number of genes over time. It is this trace and the interactions between genes over time which is of interest for a number of reasons. First, genes involved with cellular processes and disease are not being expressed in a vacuum; they are constantly interacting with each other in the cell and the answers to many of the biological questions posed by microarrays will undoubtedly lie in these interactions. Second, because of these interactions, taking a single expression measurement at a particular moment in time as the basis for a study will not necessarily yield the required results, since the gene expression of individuals is a dynamic, not static phenomenon. The measurement of an individual sample over time provides us with the raw information required to decipher which genes are subsequently affecting the expression levels of other genes or even themselves. This process is not an exact science; genes expressed at one timestep have an indirect affect on others through protein production and therefore it is difficult to determine the way in which these genes interact. Add to this the fact that there could be anywhere from 100 to 30 000 genes measured over time, each with the potential to interact, and the problem becomes very difficult indeed. Essentially the desired outcome is for the GA to arrive at a network of genetic interactions between genes in adjacent timesteps. This can be best visualized by a set of rules, for instance:

If gene_X_at_Time0 is ON THEN gene_Y_at_Time1 is OFF

This represents one connection of a very simple network where the gene expression values are represented as 'absent' and 'present', to use the Affymetrix[3] nomenclature, and only one gene affects one other. What is important is that the rule has an element (the antecedent) which relates a time in the past to a subsequent timestep (the consequent). This rule structure must be used if a causal model is to be discovered through temporal regulation. When rules have been discovered for every gene in a particular experiment, a network can be created to link genes in one timestep to the next. This network can be said to have been 'reverse engineered' from the data. That is, the actual processes of genetic interaction have been extracted from biological observation and data in the form of a network. Once a network has been extracted, this constitutes a hypothesis concerning the routes that can be taken through the network

---

[3] For more information see http://www.affymetrix.com.

so that the activity of genes in a subsequent timestep can be said to be explained by the activity of genes in a previous timestep.

Computational Complexity

This problem, however, becomes more complicated when considering true genetic interactivity as a number of genes can affect any number of genes in the next timestep, i.e. not all interactions are one-to-one. This is where GA approaches can be applied, as the number of possible networks is huge with respect to the number of genes. The fact that genes can act in combination to affect combinations of genes at the next timestep means that the problem requires the algorithm to determine a combination of N genes from the total number for each influenced gene. The following expression determines the number of combinations when choosing k individuals from a total number N

$$\frac{N!}{k!(N-k)!} \tag{8.1}$$

So all the combinations of selecting five (k) elements from a total of 10 (N) is 252. That is, if the data consists of measurements of 10 genes and we assume that only five genes at one timestep affect a gene at the next timestep, there are 252 possible combinations. Select five from 100, though, and the number of possible combinations rises to 75 287 520; select five from 10 000 (a typical gene expression experiment) and the numbers become unmanageable. The total number of solutions cannot be searched exhaustively to guarantee optimality. This problem is therefore very difficult to solve with traditional methods and this is where GAs can be used.

Graph and matrix representations

The gene regulatory network can be represented as a set of weights connecting genes in one timestep with genes in another. This matrix of weighted connections determines the effect that each gene in one timestep has on another gene in the next timestep. Figure 8.9 shows a typical genetic network and its weight matrix representation (see also Table 3.1).

It is in this way that a matrix can represent a gene regulatory network. However, Figure 8.9 shows two connections into G4, from G2 and G3.

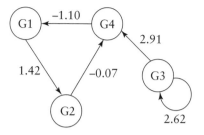

	G1	G2	G3	G4
G1	– –	– –	– –	–1.10
G2	1.42	– –	– –	– –
G3	– –	– –	2.62	– –
G4	– –	–0.07	2.91	– –

Figure 8.9   Graph and matrix representation of a gene regulatory network, where columns specify the start point and rows the end point; so, for instance, G4 influences G1 with value –1.10 (a negative gene effect)

The question of how these values can be combined to give the correct expression value of G4 remains. One approach is due to Weaver *et al.* (1999), who combined the values together and passed them through the sigmoid function (see the Chapter 7 for more on this function) to give the output for G4. Therefore, any algorithm wishing to discover a gene regulatory network must discover the set of weights that connect genes in one timestep to those in the next. These weights, combined with the expression values of the incoming genes and passed through the sigmoid function, give the required expression levels for the output gene.

Evolutionary approaches to the reverse engineering problem

A succession of papers (Ando and Iba, 2001a, 2001b) have described methods of using GAs to extract the gene regulatory networks from gene expression data. Mostly, they used the approach detailed above by Weaver, *et al.* (1999) as the model for forward activation and reverse engineering their gene regulatory networks. The GA is applied to the problem in a number of ways, in adding noise to the reverse engineering process for example, but the results most often reported refer to the following representation of the network to the GA. The chromosome of the GA is encoded as a matrix of floating point values which correspond to the weight matrix between gene timesteps (as in Figure 8.9). The fitness function for the GA is calculated as the sum, over all timesteps, of the difference between the predicted and actual level of activation for the gene expression. The GA is then allowed to optimize this matrix of weights for these criteria.

Another objective which is factored into the fitness function is that sparse matrices are required in this problem to remove the possibility of all genes having an effect on all other genes. A measure of the number of zero weights present in the chromosome is added so an individual solution fitness is based both on its solution and number of zeroes in the solution. The advantages of this process are that the GA uses Weaver *et al.*'s established method of gene regulatory network modelling and also makes use of the reverse engineering process to a certain extent. The results on artificial data are encouraging and suggest that the GA should be able to extract matrix-type gene regulatory networks from this type of data.

There are, however, some difficulties with this approach. For instance, the chromosome has to evolve the entire weight matrix for a set of genes and so the chromosome will consist of a large number of floating point values. Although this GA approach is good for modest numbers of genes, the number of interactions required in the matrix quickly become unmanageable. A network of 1000 genes possesses 1000^2 possible connections and therefore the complexity of generating networks of this size for each individual in the population is too great. The GA has no theoretical limits on the size of the chromosome that can be optimized, but there are often practical limits concerning the memory of the computer and the time taken to evaluate each chromosome on the data. Also, whilst any gene in the network *can* effect any other, the vast majority do not. Biological experimentation (Thieffry *et al.*, 1998) and chaos theory (Kauffman, 1996) suggest that the number of genes which can act together to alter the expression values of another gene (the K-value) is small (less than six). Therefore the problem size for 1000 genes is closer to $6*1000$ than $1000*1000$. To take advantage of this fact, a modified GA example (Keedwell and Narayanan, 2003) uses the GA to discover one single column of the matrix at a time. The genes affecting a gene in the next timestep are limited by the K-value, so only a handful of genes must be discovered for each optimization. The chromosome therefore has to change from a matrix representation to one which specifies the incoming gene and its weight, as shown in Figure 8.10. The GA is then run for each output gene, building up the network step by step. This representation

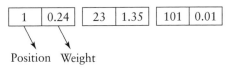

Position Weight

Figure 8.10   Gene and weight pairs chromosome representation of a gene regulatory network

reduces the computational complexity of the problem and also breaks the problem into smaller pieces, thereby allowing each element to be solved more quickly.

This is a good illustration of the importance of a good representation for solving a task with a GA. By using the known biological constraints of the problem, and by making the problem to be solved by the GA simpler, the GA can be applied to real-world gene expression data in addition to artificial problems.

Multiple sequence alignment

The task of comparing sequences is at the heart of bioinformatics. By comparing sequences of nucleic or amino acids, the similarity in structure between genes and proteins can be discovered. The ability to match two or more sequences according to the elements within those sequences is an extremely important one in bioinformatics as it allows new genes and proteins to be accurately compared with existing ones for which the structure and function are known. The comparison of these sequences can help in the discovery of similar genes across species and also help determine the phylogeny of those species. As pointed out in Chapter 2, the comparison of even two sequences is not simple. A very simple method would be to write down both sequences and compare those elements which are similar and those which are not. For instance:

```
A   C   G   C
A   T   G   C
*       *   *
```

The * character indicates a matched column between the two sequences. However, if one character is inserted or deleted, the sequence alignment no longer exists and two highly similar sequences have no matches.

```
A   C   G   C   –
–   A   T   G   C
```

The task is to determine the optimal alignment of these sequences by correctly inserting gaps to realign the sequences. Whilst the problem seems relatively trivial when only four bases and one gap is considered, the task becomes very difficult when the number of bases in a typical gene is taken into account. There are a number of algorithms which perform very well on a problem such as this with just two sequences, but multiple sequence alignment requires this process to occur for a large number of sequences. It is for this problem that researchers have turned to intelligent methods to perform this sequence alignment. Genetic algorithms in particular have been successful in this domain, pioneered by the Sequence Alignment Genetic Algorithm (SAGA) (Notredame and Higgins, 1996).

The GA approach makes use of a population of alignments where each alignment is assessed as to its performance in terms of the number of columns which match and the number of gaps which are introduced into the sequences. The genetic algorithm itself is modified from a standard algorithm in that it uses an elitist approach where 50 per cent of the best performing alignments are copied to the next generation. 22 problem-specific operators are also used. The 22 include 19 mutation operators and three cross-over operators which have to be specifically designed to modify the alignment of sequences in a meaningful way. The one-point cross-over operator, for instance, takes two separate alignments, makes a cut at a random point in the first alignment sequence and cuts the second alignment at such a point that every sequence is cut adjacent to the same symbol as in the first alignment. The left side of one parent is then spliced to the right side of the other and vice versa, and then gaps are added to ensure alignment consistency. The results taken from Notredame and Higgins (1996) show that the genetic algorithm discovered alignments that performed as well as or better than two established methods, MSA and Clustal.

The GA approach broadly described here provides a good example of the modifications that can be made to an algorithm to make use of an evolutionary approach. The representation of the problem is reasonably fixed, alignments can only be made by inserting gaps in a sequence, and the cross-over and mutation operators had to be modified accordingly. It also shows a good application of GAs to a fundamental problem in bioinformatics.

Conclusion

This section has shown a GA applied to two problems taken from bioinformatics. Each example highlights an important aspect of applying GAs to bioinformatics, namely that the correct representation and objective function can yield a very successful application. These examples also illustrate the diversity of applications of GAs, and they remain one of the best performing as well as the most flexible of the AI algorithms used for bioinformatics.

8.6 Summary of chapter

1 Genetic algorithms (GAs) make use of biologically inspired operators of *selection, cross-over* and *mutation* to move from one solution to the next, and are an efficient method of searching large spaces that are not amenable to traditional algorithms.

2 Multi-objective GAs have yet to be widely exploited in bioinformatics, but offer the researcher a set of possible solutions rather than just one and are based on the principle of dominance.

3 Genetic algorithms have been used for a number of problems in bioinformatics including the reverse engineering problem and sequence alignment.

4 The single most important element of applying a GA to a problem, regardless of domain, is to ensure that the representation of the problem to the algorithm is as close to the real problem as possible.

8.7 References and further reading

Ando, S. and Iba, H. (2001a) Inference of gene regulatory model by genetic algorithms, in *Proceedings of Conference on Evolutionary Computation 2001*, pp. 712–719.

Ando, S. and Iba, H. (2001b) The matrix modeling of gene regulatory networks – reverse engineering by genetic algorithms, in *Proceedings of Atlantic Symposium on Computational Biology, and Genome Information Systems and Technology 2001*.

Deb. K., Pratap, A., Agarwal, S. *et al.* (2000) A fast and elitist multi-objective genetic algorithm – NSGA-II *KanGAL Report Number 2000001*.

Goldberg, D.E. (1989) *Genetic Algorithms in Search Optimization and Machine Learning*. Addison Wesley.

Fogel, G.B. and Corne, D.W. (eds) (2003) *Evolutionary Computation in Bioinformatics*, Morgan Kaufmann.

Fonseca, C.M. and Fleming, P.J. (1995) An overview of evolutionary algorithms in multiobjective optimisation. *Evolutionary Computation*, 3(1), 1–16.

Holland, J.H. (1975) *Adaptation in Natural and Artificial Systems*. Ann Arbor, The University of Michigan Press.

Kauffman, S. (1996) *At Home in the Universe: The Search for Laws of Self-Organization and Complexity*. Penguin Books.

Keedwell, E.C. and Narayanan, A. (2003) Genetic algorithms for gene expression analysis. *Applications of Evolutionary Computing LNCS 2611* (eds. Gunther

Raidl *et al.*) Proceedings of EvoBIO2003 1st European Workshop on Evolutionary Bioinformatics, pp. 76–86.

Notredame, C. and Higgins, D.H. (1996) SAGA: Sequence alignment by genetic algorithm. *Nucleic Acids Res.*, **24**, 1515–24.

Thieffry, D., Huerta, A.M., Perez-Rueda, E. *et al.* (1998) From specific gene regulation to genomic networks: a global analysis of transcriptional regulation in *Escherichia coli. BioEssays Vol 20*, John Wiley and Sons Inc., New York, pp. 433–440.

Weaver, D.C., Workman, C.T. and Stormo, G.D. (1999) Modelling regulatory networks with weight matrices. *Pacific Symposium on Biocomputing*, **4**, 112–123.

Part 3
Future Techniques

9

Genetic Programming

9.1 Method

Genetic programming (GP) is one of the most recent techniques in artificial intelligence and is closely related to the GA (described in Chapter 8). It makes use of some properties of GAs in that it is a stochastic, population-based, evolutionary approach to search and optimization. However, it differs significantly from the GA in some of the operators that are used and, most crucially, in the representation of a solution to the algorithm. Traditional GAs derive a solution to a problem where the solution is represented by a string of variables (chromosome, see Chapter 8) related to the problem at hand. Genetic programming, however, uses a tree (often known as a parse tree) to represent a solution to the problem, and it is this which constitutes the main difference between GAs and GP. Genetic programming was originally conceived as a method for computers to program themselves ('automatic programming') by using these trees and it has been shown that the programs it derives can be used to represent a range of equations and functions which are based on the tree representation. Genetic programming has found a range of applications in science and engineering disciplines, most successfully in electronic circuit board design and automated programming tasks. In recent times, the founder of GP, John Koza, has been advocating the fact that GP techniques can create human-competitive designs for these and other problems. The algorithm has been able to recreate a large number of designs which were previously granted patents and some new designs that are expected to be of patentable quality. This shows the

Intelligent Bioinformatics   Edward Keedwell and Ajit Narayanan
© 2005 John Wiley & Sons, Ltd

ability of the technique to develop new solutions to problems. In addition to this, it also shows that the inventions it arrives at are very similar to those developed by humans, and lays a good claim to the name of artificial *intelligence*. As an extremely powerful technique, GP could easily be one of the most used techniques in bioinformatics in the coming years.

The algorithm

Genetic programming uses the same principles as other evolutionary techniques, in that it makes use of a population of solutions to the problem which are then manipulated by operators such as selection, mutation and crossover. These operators are executed on the population repeatedly to achieve better solutions over time. It differs, however, in the type of operators used and, as previously discussed, the representation. The following sections describe the tree representation and the operators used to create new trees during the algorithm run.

Tree representation

A tree consists of two types of elements, operators (which are distinct from the genetic operators we have seen previously) and terminals. As their name suggests operators perform operations on the terminals and terminals are essentially variables in a computer program. Common operators include the mathematical operators such as plus, minus and multiply which have arity 2 (they require two terminals to operate on) and log10, exp and square root those which have arity 1 (they require only one terminal). The terminal set consists of variables relating to the problem and also constants such as integers and real values (perhaps *PI* or *e*). The selection of operators and terminals depends very much on the problem at hand, in much the same way that the choice of decision variables is very important for the operation of GAs. A tree can be created from the operator and terminal set according to a set of simple rules.

1 The first node must be an operator.

2 An operator must have exactly the number of arguments as determined by its arity.

3 An operator can take any operator (including itself) or any terminal as an argument.

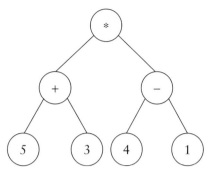

Figure 9.1 A small parse tree using the integers one to two and the standard mathematical operators; the result of this tree can be computed as 24 ((5 + 3)*(4 − 1))

Figure 9.1 shows an example tree which could be created from simple mathematical operators and the integers one to five. The initialization process of each solution must be completed in such a way that completely new, random trees are created for each individual in the population. The way in which the tree is created can be completed in a number of ways, although the most commonly used methods are 'grow' and 'full'.

1 *Grow* – In this mode, the first node is an operator, and then elements randomly taken from the complete set (terminals and operators) are added to the tree. Once the tree has reached the maximum depth (specified as a parameter), or if all operators have terminals, then the function is stopped. This process can be seen in Figure 9.2.

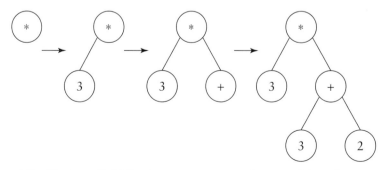

Figure 9.2 The 'grow' initialization operator – note that at each iteration any operator or terminal can be added to the tree and that the resulting tree does not necessarily have an even number of leaves; the result of this tree can be computed as 15 (3*(3 + 2)

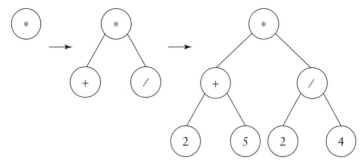

Figure 9.3 The 'full' initialization operator with maximum depth 2 – at each iteration, the operator checks to see whether it has met the maximum depth,
if so, then terminals are added, if not, then operators are added; this
tree therefore is symmetrical and its result can be computed as 3.5 ((2 +
5)*(2/4))

2 *Full* – In full mode, the first node is again an operator, but only
operators are randomly added until the maximum depth is reached.
Once this has been completed, terminals are added to the final level
of operators until they all have the required number of arguments.
This process can be seen in Figure 9.3.

The advantage of the 'grow' method is that it tends to be quicker
than the 'full' method, but the trees are usually not symmetrical and,
despite the maximum depth setting, in the worst case it is possible for
a tree which is grown to have only one operator (the initial operator).
The 'full' method takes longer to initialize than the 'grow' method but
trees of a guaranteed size (determined by the maximum depth) can be
created.

Fitness evaluation

Once a population of trees has been created, they can be evaluated for fitness in a similar way to a GA. There is a significant difference, however, in
that whereas a GA chromosome is evaluated simply by viewing the gene
values, a tree must be executed to give a result. This result can be a single
value, or it can consist of a set of values created by executing the tree
on a variety of different variable (terminal) settings. The result or results
from the tree are compared with the required result by the user-defined
objective function. The objective function therefore uses this comparison function and returns a fitness for the solution. Once the evaluation
process has been completed, the genetic operators are used to create new

solutions for the algorithm to progress to the next generation. In other words, if the user can specify *what* is required of a program and specify this requirement in the objective function, GP can be used to generate a tree (program) that describes *how* to produce what is required. So while both GAs and GP deal with solutions to problems, they differ in what they produce. Genetic algorithms produce solutions that contain combinations of parameter values (possibly weighted) to satisfy a function, whereas GP produces solutions that contain a series of instructions for producing desired and specified program behaviour.

Selection

The selection processes for GP are essentially the same as those used for GAs. The selector is only concerned with the fitness of the solution in comparison with others in the population and therefore many of the same techniques can be taken from GAs. The GA selection techniques can be seen in Chapter 8.

Crossover

Whilst GA selectors can be used for GP, the crossover operator must take into account the tree structure of the chromosome. The actual operation of the crossover remains similar in that it aims to share the genetic information of two individuals, by cutting two individuals at a certain point and exchanging genetic information at those points. However, the GP crossover must take into account the fact that operators must have the required number of terminals to operate correctly. This is achieved by guaranteeing that the crossover location in both chromosomes corresponds to a sub-tree in each individual. A sub-tree is defined as a portion of one of the main trees which could be correctly executed on its own, i.e. that all the operators have the correct number of terminals. The steps in this crossover are:

1   choose a random point on the chromosome;

2   evaluate whether this point is the start of a sub-tree – if not, return to 1;

3   execute 1–2 on the second chromosome;

4   swap the subtrees.

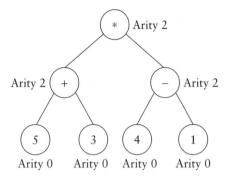

Polish notation*	*	+	5	3	–	4	1
Arity	2	2	0	0	2	0	0
Z value (arity – 1)	1	1	–1	–1	1	–1	–1
Cumulative Z value	1	2	1	0	1	0	–1
Sub-tree found	No	No	No	No	No	No	Yes

*The process of converting a tree to polish notation can be seen in figure 9.5.

Figure 9.4   Detecting sub-trees for crossover

The vital point here is step 2, determining whether the random point is the start of a sub-tree. To discover this, once the random point is determined, the algorithm moves along the tree, maintaining a sum Z. As the algorithm moves along the tree, if an operator is encountered, its arity minus one is added to Z. Terminals cannot take arguments and have an arity of zero, therefore if a terminal is encountered, 1 is removed from the total Z. If Z reaches the value of -1, a sub-tree has been located and the start and end points of the sub-tree can be recorded. This process is shown in Figure 9.4 and locates potential sub-trees from any point on the chromosome. The calculations in Figure 9.4 show that the sub-tree is identified by a -1 result by progressing through the tree maintaining a sum (-1) of the arity of any operators. Terminals cannot take any arguments (they have zero arity), and therefore they are represented as 0 in the calculation. If the result is not -1 then the resulting tree is not a sub-tree and cannot be used for crossover. Other methods exist to discover crossover points, but this is one of the most intuitive. A further example is to start at the plus operator, so $2 = 1$, then add terminal 5 $(2 = 0)$ and terminal 3 $(2 = -1)$. This also constitutes a valid subtree.

Mutation

Mutation in GP is also different from that in GAs, again due to the maintenance of tree structure. In GAs, mutation can occur by simply changing one bit in the chromosome. In GP this can also be accomplished by changing one bit, but operators must be mutated to other operators and likewise with terminals. If this principle is violated, the structure of the tree breaks down and a syntactically invalid tree can be created.

Another method is to use the technique developed in the initialization to create new sub-trees in the tree. The process for this is shown:

1 select a random point X on the tree;

2 if X is an operator, go to 3 otherwise repeat 1;

3 delete the sub-tree leading from X, and add a new sub-tree using either the 'grow' or 'full' method of initialization described earlier.

This process leads to substantially new material being added to the tree and therefore constitutes an effective mutation technique.

With the application of standard selection, and specific mutation and crossover (of which only a few examples are seen here) operators, new, better-performing trees can be created to solve a large variety of problems.

Tree interpretation

Whilst the above algorithm is well formulated in terms of the manipulation of trees, the question remains as to why trees should be created at all. A tree differs from a traditional GA approach in that the actual variables of the problem only form a subset of the total structure used by the algorithm. The tree notion is usually used to represent an equation or function, where problem variables are combined with a variety of operators to arrive at a single representation that solves the problem. For example, if we wanted an equation to result in the number 43 using only the integers 1 to 5 and the common mathematical operators, GP could find the combination of operators to accomplish this. Once a tree has been created, it can be converted into a normal mathematical or programming language format so that it can be read and verified intuitively. Also there are some programming languages, such as Lisp and other functional and logic programming languages, that use tree structures for representing both data and function. If GP is implemented in these languages, there is a natural way of executing the tree structures within these languages through the use of an 'evaluation' command on a tree. Figures 9.1, 9.2 and 9.3 illustrate this process.

Polish notation

In many GP applications, trees are expressed in Polish notation or reverse Polish notation. Polish notation was devised by the Polish philosopher and mathematician Jan Lucasiewicz (1878–1956). This notation allows a two-dimensional tree to be represented as a string of characters and converted easily back to the tree format. The recursive nature of converting trees can appear complex at first, but a number of steps executed repeatedly allows this conversion to take place. Figure 9.5 shows the process of converting a tree into Polish notation and back again. The order in which elements of the tree are added to the string are shown next to each element of the tree. Each element is added depth first, until a terminal is encountered. Once an operator has all its arguments, the process moves back up the tree and fills those operators that still have unfilled arguments.

The rule is that the elements are added depth first, so an operator of arity 2 followed by two further operators leaves each of the operators unsatisfied. Operator 2 occupies one argument of operator 1 and operator 3 occupies only one argument of operator 2. Operator 3 has no arguments filled until further operators or terminals are added. With each successive addition of an operator or terminal, if there are no more free arguments then move back up the tree and fill operators further up. It is this recursive nature of both the creation and execution of

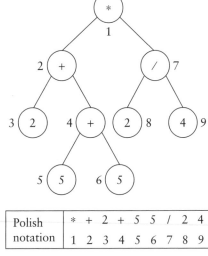

Figure 9.5   Converting parse trees to Polish notation

these trees which can be one of the more difficult concepts to grasp. By creating some simple expressions in Polish notation and writing them as trees, the method can be learnt quickly.

Bloat

Genetic programming trees are often subject to a phenomenon known as 'bloat'. By necessity, GP uses variable length chromosomes to represent trees and, theoretically at least, these trees can have infinite depth. However, in most applications a tree beyond a certain size is costly to process, unwieldy to interpret and often fails to generalize beyond the training set that it has been given. The increase of a tree size beyond a required limit (known as 'bloat') is a significant problem with GP, since the execution time for trees can increase very rapidly as they grow in depth.

There exist a number of strategies to mitigate this effect, including:

1 introduction of a fitness penalty based on the depth of the tree,

2 introduction of a hard threshold so that trees cannot exceed a certain depth,

3 multiple-objective approaches, using tree depth as a second objective (Bleuler et al., 2001).

The first strategy ensures that very large trees are unlikely to be created since the fitness will be reduced if the tree becomes large. On the other hand, a satisfactory solution (tree) may be inadvertently deleted by this strategy. The second strategy is a little more difficult to implement and ensures that computation time is strictly limited. This strategy, however, can also be problematic (like the first strategy) if very good trees for the problem tend to be large.

The final strategy does not guarantee that processing times will be small, but rather gives a set of trees which are evaluated both for their size and accuracy. Whilst limits can be placed on multi-objective approaches (by using methods such as constrained-dominance (Deb et al., 2000)), an unconstrained multi-objective approach would not remove bloat from the algorithm. The processing time would be similar to a standard GP run as solutions with higher depth would be accepted alongside smaller solutions. However, it would highlight the relationship between tree depth and accuracy and could therefore prove to be useful in determining what amount of bloat is necessary to deliver the required result accuracy. The problem of bloat is therefore significant, but a number of strategies exist in the literature to mitigate its effect.

Conclusion

Genetic programming represents one of the most powerful and flexible techniques for deriving the equations and functions about unknown systems. The properties of the GP algorithm are quite different from those of the GA and consequently less well-understood and used. The fundamental evolutionary processes that underpin the GA are maintained in GP, but the trees that are derived require special manipulation and interpretation.

The following sections describe how to implement GP for bioinformatics problems and also some existing applications of them in this field.

9.2 Application guidelines

Introduction

Genetic programming can be applied to a large number of problems and has been successfully applied in a number of areas. To a certain extent, the same application requirements for GAs apply to GP, i.e. the problem should possess an objective function that responds relatively smoothly to changes in the chromosome. The issue of problem representation is less pronounced for GP, since trees are the default representation. However, a number of parameters must be selected with care when using GP. These issues are discussed below.

Terminal selection

Genetic programming is sensitive to the type and range of variables it is given, and much thought must be given to the terminals and operators supplied to the algorithm to enable it to perform well in its task. Genetic programming can combine and recombine its problem variables in a way that GAs cannot. For instance, if GP requires the variable 0.6 in an equation, it can create this by combining the terminals 6 and 10, and the divide operator. The algorithm can overcome some shortcomings in the representation of the problem, but it will still require as many variables (terminals) relating to the problem as possible. Generally speaking, random constants are also added as terminals to allow GP a greater freedom in deriving equations. The number and range of these constants will depend on the problem itself.

Operator selection

Operator selection can be a tricky business as the more powerful operators such as power, exp, factorial, etc. can easily create numbers which are beyond the range of most personal computers. The problem is that, due to the random nature of GP, any of these operators can be applied to any other, and the same operator can even be 'nested' and applied to itself repeatedly. The following example shows two nested power operators:

$$POW(50, POW(10,2)) = POW(50, 100) = 50^{100}.$$

As can be seen, this result would be a huge number even though only the power operator and some reasonably small integers were used. Such operators must be carefully restricted or, in some cases, eliminated from GP altogether.

Aside from these unrestricted operators, there are a large number of standard mathematical functions that can be used, such as plus, minus, multiply, etc., but care must be taken with the divide function as it must be restricted so that a divide by zero error cannot occur. If either of the arguments is zero, then a zero is returned as opposed to performing the divide function. This is not a difficult fix, but does illustrate that care must be taken when devising operators for use with GP.

General applications

As with GAs, the applicability of GP to a problem will depend on whether a well-formed objective function can be created and whether the required solution can be represented as a program or function. A variety of applications and a wealth of other information can be found at John Koza's website[1]. Koza is often described as the 'father' of GP and this site describes in detail some of the more impressive feats of GP. These include 'human-competitive' applications where GP has created previously patented inventions, or new inventions which are determined to be of

---

[1] More information can be found at http://www.genetic-programming.org.

patentable quality. Through this website the power of GP, and in particular its ability to display 'human-competitive' intelligent behaviour, are illustrated.

Software

A smaller subject field than GAs, GP has fewer implementations for potential users. Generally speaking, GA software can be converted to perform GP as long as it can form variable length chromosomes. However, a large list of free and commercial be spoke GP implementations can be found at The Genetic Programming Notebook[2], the most notable of which is Discipulus[3], a commercial Windows™ package.

9.3 Bioinformatics applications

Introduction

Genetic programming has only been in existence since the early 1990s and therefore is one of the newest techniques contained in this book. Whilst this pre-dates much of the modern bioinformatics research, a number of more established techniques are often used before GP is considered. Therefore the number of GP applications to bioinformatics problems is currently small. As with other areas of science and engineering, GP is starting to make more of an impact and the work undertaken here shows the diversity of existing applications of GP to bioinformatics problems.

Genetic programming in data mining for drug discovery

This work conducted by Langdon and Barrett (2004) is a neat example of how GP can be applied to the problem of drug discovery for human medicinal purposes. Drug discovery as a whole field is a 'hot topic' in bioinformatics as currently it takes a new drug compound between 10 and 12 years to get into mainstream usage. Much of this time is often spent testing the drug firstly in the laboratory and then later in organisms

[2] More information can be found at http://www.geneticprogramming.com.
[3] More information can be found at http://www.aimlearning.com.

and animals. Whilst the laboratory testing stage of a drug is relatively cheap, it can also be frustrating as there will exist many compounds with similar properties that have to be tested. Pharmaceutical companies are constantly searching for automated methods to help them target their search in these initial stages. Langdon and Barrett showed that GP can be successfully used for determining the bioavailability of a set of compounds based on their structure. The bioavailability of a compound is one of a set of metrics and is designed to determine how well a drug will pass through the various bodily systems and, on reaching the active site, how much effect the drug will have. If taken orally, a drug is subject to many bodily mechanisms such as digestion, metabolism and excretion. Some compounds will be relatively unaffected by these processes whereas others will have practically no effect on their target because they have been broken down by these bodily functions before they can reach the target site.

Method

The task for GP is to determine which of a set of compounds will satisfy the requirements for drug bioavailability. The notion of 'acceptable' is determined by a threshold value of 33 for bioavailability with those falling below this level deemed 'poor' and those above 'acceptable'. By applying this threshold, a classification problem is created to distinguish between the poor and acceptable compounds. The classification accuracy of the system is computed as the 'ROC convex hull' approach (ROC stands for receiver operating characteristics), which is an ingenious method of giving false positives and false negatives the same importance in the fitness function. Readers are directed to Langdon and Barrett (2004) for more detail on how this works, as they demonstrate an excellent way of transforming a classification problem into a smooth objective function for use with genetic techniques. The method was trained and tested on a variety of data, taken from drug trials on both humans and rats. As would be expected, the data on rat bioavailability was more abundant and better distributed, since the human data consisted only of those drugs which made it through initial screening. Each drug compound was represented by 83 variables that were used to identify functional groups within each drug. These functional groups have been identified and developed over a long period of time by the pharmaceutical companies and included electrical, structural, topological and physico-chemical features of the compound.

In addition to the chemical variables, a variety of constants (some of which were random) were added to the terminal set. The operator set consisted of the standard mathematical operators (with a protected divide operator as discussed earlier) and a four-level 'if' conditional operator. This set of constants, operators and variables perfectly illustrates an application of GP to a bioinformatics problem. The constants and operators give the GP the flexibility to provide combinations of the feature variables, and the 'if' statement allows the algorithm additional scope to develop logical rules as well as standard equations.

Genetic programming was run on each of the datasets and tested on a hold-out dataset (to determine how well the created trees generalize beyond the training set). The performance on the human dataset was better than the performance on the rat dataset, but it was discovered that the trees discovered for the human data did not generalize to (i.e. perform well on) the rat data. However, the reverse was true: the trees generated on the admittedly larger rat dataset were successful in predicting bioavailability in the human dataset.

This finding suggests that human and rat bioavailability are closely related and, perhaps more significantly, GP discovered a set of features which was applicable to both species. The tree which correctly classified both sets of data was able to be significantly simplified with only a small loss in performance and was subsequently much simpler than expected. This not only highlighted the possibility that bioavailability was more simple than previously thought, but also shows the power of the GP approach. Whilst the constituent elements of a tree are simple operators and terminals, they can be combined together with great effect and the final trees can be easily interpreted and simplified by end-users.

Genetic programming for functional genomics in yeast data

This work, undertaken in 2000 by Gilbert, Rowland and Kell represents one of the first applications of GP to a bioinformatics topic. This research used some of the first reliable gene expression data taken from a set of experiments with a species of yeast, *Saccharomyces cerevisiae*. The data itself was collected in a time-course experiment where the yeast was exposed to a set of 79 different experimental conditions, including heat shock, reducing shock and sporulation (for more on this see Eisen *et al.*, 1998). Each of the genes had been assigned one of six classes – 'Histone', 'Proteasome', 'TCA Pathway', 'Respiratory Complex', 'Ribosome' and

'HTH-containing' – which were learnt from existing functional knowledge. The task for GP was to assign genes to the correct classes using their gene expression profiles over the 79 experiments.

Method

Each gene was represented by a set of expression values over time and was added to the dataset of some 304 training genes and 152 testing genes. The objective function was to minimize the number of classification errors determined by the rules where each individual in the population comprised six rules (one for each class). Therefore a single individual in the population could classify the entire training set of genes, by utilizing its six rules to determine to which class the gene belongs. If a gene was found which did not trigger the execution of any of the rules, it was assumed that that gene had an unknown function. To accomplish this task, the GP implementation used the standard set of mathematical operators, and an 'if greater than or equal to operator' which compared two variables and returned a one for true, or zero for false.

This GP implementation was run five times on this problem (with different random seeds) and the results were very encouraging. The method correctly classified the vast majority of the training and test data, returning 100 per cent test accuracy on the classes Histone, TCA Pathway and Respiratory Complex. The three remaining classes were classified with a maximum of two misclassifications on the test data. In 80% of runs the GP discovered the rule *if alpha [35] ≥ alpha [49] then "TCA Pathway" else "Unknown"*, suggesting that all the TCA pathway genes can be identified using just the 35 minute and 49 minute timepoints from the α-factor cell division cycle experiment. This shows that the GP approach can be used to classify genes successfully by functionality based on their expression levels across experiments. In addition to this, the authors applied the classifier to the entire dataset and found that some 291 genes were predicted to be of class *ribosome* (characterised by the rule *if (elution [30] − leaf [20] − diauxic [b]) ≥ (alpha [119] + 1.15335) then "Ribosome" else "Unknown")*). Of these 291, 121 had previously been identified as ribosomal genes, and the remaining 170 had known or suspected function. Of these 170, 102 of the genes appeared to have functionally-similar properties to ribosomal genes. The authors therefore surmised that the current classification schema for these genes was too strict, and that the GP approach had found a more inclusive system for classifying these genes. A further important attribute of this approach was that the GP trees, once converted into rules, could then easily be interpreted by biologists and assessed for their biological feasibility. This transparency was often not present in other classification methods, such as neural networks and other clustering techniques. The application of GP here was therefore vital in the further understanding of the yeast gene expression data due to its ability to extract meaningful and accurate information from the data.

Therefore this approach shows all the desirable features of the GP algorithm. The approach was firstly able to classify correctly the set of genes on which it was trained, and also test data that was not part of the training process. In addition to this, the classifier was used on the entire dataset to predict a certain classification for a number of genes, a number of which agreed with a current functional genomic database, and a number of which appeared to have similar function. Finally, the approach was able to identify the genes used in the classifier in an easily-digestible manner and this led to the proposed classification of a number of previously functionally-unknown genes. This work therefore demonstrates the power, flexibility and accuracy of the GP approach.

9.4 Background

The basis of GP was formed with the discovery of GAs by John Holland (see Chapter 8 for more on this), as this laid the foundations for evolved population search. The subsequent discovery of GP is often attributed to John Koza (1992) who first arrived at the idea of evolving programs rather than strings of bits and other more static representations. Since this time, there has been a steady increase in the number of researchers working with GP, but the field is still much smaller than that of the GA.

9.5 Summary of chapter

1 Genetic programming is one of the family of evolutionary techniques that include GAs. They operate broadly in the same fashion in that they use a population of solutions, stochastic operators and an objective function.

2 They differ from GAs in that they evolve parse trees from operators and terminals rather than a static set of variables. To accomplish this, the chromosome needs to be of variable length.

3 Genetic programming trees can suffer from bloat, be expressed in Polish notation and can often be extensively simplified from their evolved state.

4 Genetic programming has discovered human-competitive patentable inventions and has also found applications in many areas of science and engineering, including bioinformatics

9.6 References

Bleuler, S., Brack, M., Thiele, L. *et al.* (2001) *Multiobjective Genetic Programming: Reducing Bloat Using SPEA2*. Proceedings of Congress on Evolutionary Computation (CEC 2001), pp. 536–543.

Deb, K., Agrawal, S., Pratap, A. *et al.* (2000). *A Fast Elitist Non-dominated Sorting Genetic Algorithm for Multi-objective Optimization: NSGA-II*. Proceedings of the Parallel Problem Solving from Nature VI Conference , 16–20 September. (Paris, France), pp. 849–858.

Eisen, M.B., Spellman, P.T., Brown, P.O. *et al.* (1998) Cluster analysis and display of genome-wide expression patterns *Proc. Natl. Acad. Sci.*, **95**, 14863–14868.

Gilbert, R.J, Rowland, J.J. and Kell, D.B. (2000) Genomic computing: explanatory modelling for functional genomics, in *Proceedings of the Genetic and Evolutionary Computation Conference (GECCO-2000)* (eds D. Whitley *et al.*, July 10–12, 2000), Las Vegas, Nevada, USA. Morgan Kaufmann, pp. 551–557.

Koza, J.R. (1992) *Genetic Programming: On the Programming of Computers by Means of Natural Selection*. MIT Press, Cambridge, Massachusetts.

Langdon, W.B. and Barrett, S.J. (2004) Genetic programming in data mining for drug discovery in *Evolutionary Computing in Data Mining*, (eds A. Ghosh and L.C. Jain), Physica Verlag, pp. 211–235.

10

Cellular Automata

10.1 Method

Cellular automata (CA) are unlike many of the other techniques presented in this book in that they are more often used for the simulation and modelling of systems rather than for optimization or classification. This is largely due to the fact that they were originally conceived to simulate complex systems arising in nature such as those seen in physics, chemistry or biology. In all these examples, the systems are complex because of the interactions of a number of elements contained within a fixed environment. In chemistry and physics, molecules and atoms collide and react with each other countless times a second, and in biology small organisms such as bacteria compete with each other for resources. The common thread to all these systems is that individual elements, be they molecules, atoms or organisms, interact with each other *in parallel*. Traditional serial models of computation can make these interactions difficult to calculate, but CA represent an alternative to this because they can model these large-scale interactions between elements in a parallel fashion. This is possible because CA consist of a uniform grid of cells, each of which can be thought of as a point of space. Each of the cells contains a small number of bits of information which represent the *state* of that cell. The state of each cell is updated by using rules (known as state transition rules) which, based on the states of other neighbouring cells, change the state of the current cell accordingly. The state transition rules themselves must be uniformly applied across the whole grid of cells. This approach enables a rudimentary simulation of systems with multiple

Intelligent Bioinformatics   Edward Keedwell and Ajit Narayanan
© 2005 John Wiley & Sons, Ltd

elements, since each cell can be occupied by one of the elements by a modification of its state (at its most simple, occupied or not-occupied). In this fashion two adjacent occupied elements can be thought of as 'reacting' or 'colliding'. The state transition rules then determine what occurs when two adjacent cells are occupied and what occurs to the elements once they have reacted. It is in this way that a contained 'universe' can be simulated by using CA and in the past, parallels have been drawn between CA and a stylized universe operating under a set of uniform laws. Cellular automata can therefore be useful in modelling physical systems including diffusion, fluid dynamics, ballistic computation, chemical reactions and biological phenomena.

They are often difficult techniques to apply in many areas, including bioinformatics, as special attention must be paid towards the system formulation. The system must be separable into the discrete elements seen in a CA, or of course represented in such a way that this level of granularity is acceptable. Once this has been accomplished, CA offer a type of computation to different from any of the other techniques described in this book, with the opportunity of simulating complex systems in an efficient fashion. The following sections describe the basic operation of a CA and some potential applications of the technique.

The grid of cells

As described previously, a CA consists of a grid of cells which can adopt a number of states. In the most simple example, each cell can adopt one of two states (on or off, 1 or 0), but some applications as will be seen later require a significantly greater number than this. Each cell has a neighbourhood of additional cells which surround it in the grid the definition of which is important in the execution of the state transition rules. Figure 10.1 gives an example of some different neighbourhoods. The black

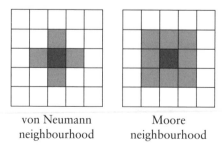

von Neumann
neighbourhood

Moore
neighbourhood

Figure 10.1 Two possible neighbourhoods for use in a CA

square represents the cell under consideration and the shaded squares correspond to the neighbours of that cell. A von Neumann neighbourhood allows cells to communicate with up, down, left and right cells. A Moore neighbourhood, on the other hand, contains the von Neumann neighbourhood plus the diagonally contiguous cells. These are just two examples, there are many other neighbourhoods, especially when three- and higher-dimensional CA are considered.

The state of each cell is influenced by the states of cells within the specified neighbourhood. It is in this way that the selection of the neighbourhood influences the path that the cellular automaton will take. Neighbourhood selection is highly dependent on the problem domain that the automaton is intending to simulate. In some applications, reactions can take place over some distance, whereas in others the elements must be adjacent to be able to react. The state transition rules take into account the number and type of elements in the neighbourhood of the current cell and so are often designed with the neighbourhood in mind.

State transition rules

Cellular automata are executed in discrete timesteps. The grid is 'frozen' at each timestep and the state transition rules applied to every cell in the grid before the states are updated and the rules are applied again. This discrete time behaviour is important for the control of the CA. To proceed from one step to the next, a rule or set of rules is executed to determine how the state of the current cell changes with respect to its current state and of those in its neighbourhood. These rules are uniformly applied to all cells in the grid and therefore direct the computation of the CA. However, no update of cells is allowed in most CA until and unless all cells have applied their transition rules. When they have, all the updates will be flushed through the CA to result in a new configuration. The process is iterative and is applied for as long as the CA is allowed to run.

Conway's life

One of the most elegant and simple examples of a CA is 'life' designed by John Conway. The state transition rule-set is simple, but shows a 'glider' phenomenon which represents an emergent property. These emergent properties are high-level concepts that are the result of applying rules at a local level. In 'life' a single object is seen to move or 'glide' across the screen, but this is actually only the result of applying simplistic rules to each of the cells which make up the grid in which the glider is seen. The rule-set for 'life' and an illustration of the glider phenomenon are shown below.

1   If a cell is off (state 0) and exactly three of its neighbours are on (state 1) then that cell becomes on (state 1) in the next timestep, otherwise it remains off.

2   If a cell is on and either two or three of its neighbours are on, then in the next timestep, that cell remains on, otherwise it is turned off.

Figure 10.2 shows how a simple set of rules, when applied repeatedly, can achieve an emergent phenomenon. In this case the object in the top-left corner appears to glide down and to the right with every four timesteps of the CA execution. The rules themselves are designed to represent (very loosely) life and death in a set of organisms and work thus. A

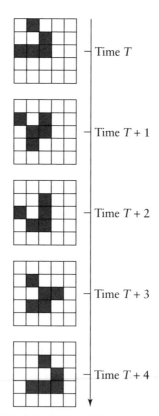

Figure 10.2   A graphical depiction of Conway's 'life' application of CA

cell which is on is occupied by an organism, and when three individuals surround it, a new organism is born. To survive, an organism needs a certain number of other organisms surrounding it (in this case two or three), otherwise it dies from exposure or overcrowding. This example provides a rudimentary example of how principles can be taken from biology and loosely applied to the CA approach. These rules represent only one form of 'life', a huge number of others can be seen on the internet[1]. What is interesting is that the behaviour observed – that of a five-cell organism gliding one-step south-east – is an emergent property that could not have been predicted from a knowledge of the transition rules alone. That is, the property emerges only for certain initial configurations, and there is nothing in the rules that tells us which configurations will display a gliding move and which other configurations will not. The only way to find out is to run the CA for different initial configurations and see what happens.

There are numerous rule-sets that can be created simply with a two-dimensional automaton and neighbourhood pairing. This, when combined with more complex states, can yield a wide variety of behaviours and application possibilities. However, it is the richness of state transition rules which give CA their flexibility and power. Toffoli and Margolus (1987) describe a set of principles which can be used to extend the capability of state transition rules.

1 *Second-order rules* – These rules use the historic state behaviour of cells (both the current cell and neighbourhood cells) to compute a new state for the current cell. This allows the automaton to use some short-term memory in its decision making.

2 *Probabilistic rules* – With these rules, state changes are executed according to a probability. In contrast to the rules described thus far, a probabilistic rule could, given the same state, choose from a number of state changes based on their probability. The advantages of this type of rule would be that the CA behaves in a more stochastic, rather than deterministic, manner.

By increasing the complexity and variety of the state transition rules, a large number of applications of CA are possible. The types of rules suggested above add depth to the approach by incorporating time as a third dimension. This can yield more complex and realistic simulations

---

[1] For some excellent illustrations of other types of 'life' see http://www.math.com/students/wonders/life/life.html.

of systems that depend not only on the current state of the system, but the state of the system in some previous generation. It is also possible to increase the dimensions of the grid itself, yielding three-dimensional systems or even four-dimensional when time is considered.

Given a CA, a set of rules and a neighbourhood, the algorithm or simulation can be run for a predetermined number of iterations. However, the behaviour of the CA, given this information, cannot be predicted in advance. The algorithm must be run to determine its behaviour and therefore its classification. Wolfram (1984) identified four classes of CA depending on their behaviour.

Class 1. After a finite number of timesteps, the CA tends to achieve a unique state (limit point) from nearly all possible starting conditions.

Class 2. The CA creates patterns that repeat periodically or are stable (limit cycles).

Class 3. From nearly all starting conditions, the CA leads to aperiodic-chaotic patterns (that is patterns that repeat without any specific period), where the statistical properties of these patterns are almost identical after a sufficient period of time to the starting patterns, thereby producing self-similar fractal curves.

Class 4. After a finite number of steps, the CA usually dies, but there are a few stable (periodic) patterns possible.

The 'life' game described earlier certainly falls into Class 2 and possibly into Class 4, since the initial configuration leads to periodically repeating patterns that have moved across the grid.

Conclusions

The theory of CA of discrete cells and universally applied rules remains the same for each application, but the actual execution of the algorithm differs considerably depending on the type of problem. Until recently CA were considered interesting from a purely theoretical point of view, although they are starting to find more practical applications, including in bioinformatics. The only restrictions on the technique are that to qualify as a CA the following elements must be satisfied.

1   The rules must be locally orientated and must be applied uniformly across the automaton.

2   Each cell must contain only a few bits of data and consist of a finite number of states.

3   Time must advance in discrete steps.

Often the problem definition determines the number of states, the transition rules and any emergent phenomena which arise from executing the automaton. The CA approach can be useful in a number of applications, as will be shown later, and can reward the extra effort required to code the problem in this format.

10.2 Application guidelines

Introduction

As described previously, the number of CA applications to real-world science and engineering problems is relatively few. Instead of solving problems or optimizing biological systems that are the focus of many of the other intelligent techniques in this book, CA have largely been involved in the simulation of physical systems. They have also been studied for their emergent and chaotic properties and, while interesting from a theoretical viewpoint, these studies can be difficult to apply to the real world. However, optimization and simulation can be accomplished with CA given the correct problem formulation due to the inherent flexibility in the creation of rule-sets. Therefore the majority of time should be spent converting the problem into a rule-set that will give the required optimization or simulation results. The following section describes a CA approach to an engineering optimization problem as the majority of the bioinformatics applications in the subsequent section are simulative in nature.

Example optimization problem

An example of a non-bioinformatics application is that of optimizing water distribution networks by using CA (Keedwell and Khu, 2004). A water distribution network contains many elements, but the simplest networks have demand nodes (vertices) and pipes connecting these nodes (edges). The aim of the optimization is to change the size of the pipes so that the demand for water at each of the nodes is met. The sizes of pipes are taken from a discrete table and have a cost associated with them. Larger pipe sizes incur increased cost, but allow more water to be delivered, whereas the reverse is true for smaller diameter pipes. To solve this problem, nodes in the network are represented by cells in the cellular automaton and can be in a deficit (not enough water) or surplus (too much water) state. There are then various rules executed which size the pipes so that the deficits and surpluses are minimized. These rules increment a pipe size if there is a deficit at the node to which it is delivering water and decrement it otherwise. This approach therefore attempts to implicitly minimize cost but maximize the delivered water. The CA starts in a random state but the rules drive it to a state of equilibrium. The early indications are that this technique can provide reasonable quality results whilst requiring only a handful of network simulations in comparison with standard GA (see Chapter 8) approaches.

This application, whilst not related to biology gives an example of how network problems can be solved by using a cellular approach. The nodes themselves do not make up a grid in a physical sense, but are all separated by at least one pipe and therefore can be seen to make up a regular grid. The node states are discrete and few, another requirement for a CA, and the fact that the optimization proceeds in discrete steps completes the set of requirements for the problem to be solved using a CA technique. Therefore even if the problem does not appear to be immediately applicable to cellular automaton optimization, it is possible that a formulation can be created if the above criteria are satisfied.

Software

Cellular automata are unlike many of the other techniques that are described elsewhere in this book because they are not generic algorithms in the same way as GAs or neural networks. Both of these techniques are reasonably generic, in that they can be applied to different problems with relatively small alterations or the tuning of some parameters. However, this is generally not the case with CA, because they rely on a set of rules which have to be problem-specific to operate. A number of software packages exist (most of them share or freeware) that offer good visualization facilities to monitor the cellular automaton as it evolves and also a framework to write rules for specific problems. Even with good software, a large amount of problem-specific coding will have to be completed within the software itself. Despite this, a good resource exists at the CelLab[2] where an online tutorial gives a good account of further theory and applications of CA and also an extensive CA framework with

---

[2] For more information go to http://www.fourmilab.ch/cellab/.

example rules and the ability to write your own rule-sets in a variety of languages. Perhaps due to this inherent problem specificity, commercial packages exploiting CA techniques are very sparse.

10.3 Bioinformatics applications

As mentioned previously, CA have found application in a number of science and engineering areas since their inception in the late 1940s. In recent times, though, they have been used in a variety of biological simulation applications where the notion is that the complex dynamical systems present in much of biology can be simplified and understood by applying discrete systems such as CA. What follows is a description of some of the most interesting work in this area using CA.

Cellular automata model for enzyme kinetics

The work undertaken by Kier *et al.* (1996) pre-dates many of the modern technological advances in bioinformatics, but it provides a simple example of how CA could be used to model a system that could be difficult to compute using standard methods. The authors use a CA approach to model the reaction between an enzyme and substrate in water. The CA consists of a 110*110 grid of cells (12 100 cells), each of which can take the values of one molecule of E (enzyme), S (substrate), P (product) and W (water); 69 per cent of the automaton was covered with water and 31 per cent was deemed to be space. When any ingredients are added, they are assumed to replace the water part of the automaton and therefore this cavity ratio was maintained. Each cell has a probability associated with its movement and its interaction with other molecules in the automaton. An enzyme molecule could react with the substrate, product and water molecules, but not with another enzyme. Molecules were determined to be adjacent according to a von Neumann neighbourhood, where the four adjoining cells (up, down, left and right) were determined to be interacting. The extended von Neumann neighbourhood increased this to two adjoining cells. The general approach to this CA can be seen in Figure 10.3. This is an extended version of the von Neumann neighbourhood shown in Figure 10.1. Note that an extra set of cells are considered with each iteration of the CA.

The affinities of certain molecules to other molecules were determined by a probability of joining, breaking and movement. An indication of the effect of the breaking parameter was exemplified in the breaking

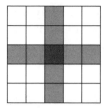

Figure 10.3   The extended von Neumann neighbourhood

probability of water molecules. The manipulation of this parameter was equivalent to manipulating the temperature of the water in which the reactions were taking place. For the following experiments, this parameter was set to replicate the temperature of the human body. Along with a parameter to determine the extent to which enzymes reacted with substrate, this completed the set of parameters required to run the CA.

Results

The CA was run with 50 enzyme cells and a variable amount of substrate for 100 iterations for each run, and was run 100 times to obtain average values for results of the runs. Initial velocities were found to vary with respect to the substrate concentration in accordance with Michaelis–Menten kinetics and generated good Lineweaver–Burke plots. In addition to this the water-like (polar) or lipophilic (non-polar) characteristics of each of the molecules varied as expected biologically by changing the pertinent parameters of the CA.

Conclusion

This work represented a significant application of CA in a biological problem environment. The automaton agreed with well-established equations for computing the reaction rates of enzymes and substrate reactions and therefore was validated as a method for simulating these reactions. However, as the authors pointed out, the replication of known variables did not advance the area of research significantly and new information must be obtained from a model for it to be successful. By varying parameters in the model, the authors were able to determine that a lower affinity between the substrate and water led to increased conversion of substrate to product. This indicated that the affinity of the substrate to water was more important than the modelled affinity between the enzyme itself and the substrate. This was a significant finding and was corroborated by further experimental results. Therefore this showed the value of an accurate CA model, in that small changes in the state transition rule parameters could manifest differences in global behaviour which were significant in the understanding of the biological system. In fact, this application showed a significant application of AI technology to a biological problem because it was found to accurately simulate the system, which could then be perturbed *in silico*. This process then led to a hypothesis which was confirmed by biological experimentation and yielded new knowledge about the process of enzyme–substrate reaction in a human-like environment.

Simulation of an apoptosis reaction network using cellular automata

To a certain extent based on the above approach, the work undertaken by Siehs *et al.* (2002) used a CA to simulate the molecular reaction pathways of apoptosis (cell death). Apoptosis is an important process in multicellular organisms since it allows cellular regeneration to take place. In addition to this, the modelling of the apoptosis process could potentially permit a greater understanding of the mechanisms of cancerous cells, since these cells are often characterized by the inhibition of the apoptosis process.

The CA itself was more complex than that seen in the previous experiment. The grid of cells was two-dimensional in nature and contained a reasonably complex data structure at each cell point. Each of these data structures consisted of a number of 'registers' which stored variables relating the current state of the molecules within the cell and its surrounds.

Register 1. The type of molecular object occupying the site. More than one object could occupy a site at a particular time.

Register 2. Reaction rate constants of each of the molecules occupying the site.

Register 3. Molecular neighbourhood (Moore neighbourhood). This stored the molecule type of each of its neighbours (up, down, left and right).

Register 4. Distribution of local momentum, based on the hard sphere collision model.

Register 5. Potential energy status of the molecules on the current site. This was computed as a function of the attraction/repulsion of molecules both on the current site and those in the neighbourhood.

Register 6. Molecular reaction lists. Determined what, if any, reaction occurred when two molecules occupied the same site.

Register 7. Reaction product lists. Determined what products occurred as a result of the reactions occurring in register 6.

Register 8. Moved direction. This register computed the location of each of the molecules at time $t + 1$ given the information in registers 4 and 5.

This CA was unusual in that each of the cells could be in a large number of states due to the combination of parameters in each of the registers. However, they were updated in discrete timesteps and based only on local information, so this implementation was still a CA. Each time the automaton was updated (the state transition rules were applied), six steps were performed as follows.

Step 1. Evaluation of molecular collisions and redistribution of kinetic energies.

Step 2. Propagation of type information from cells into register 3.

Step 3. Computation of the local potential energy situation.

Step 4. Evaluation of chemical reactions.

Step 5. Computation of the grid positions of the molecules in the next timestep.

Step 6. Full update of the grid based on computational steps 1–5.

These steps, combined with the data structure previously seen, provided a realistic model of the reaction pathways that could occur in the cell in apoptosis. This represents a complex set of states and state transition rules but crucially, due to their limited local influence and discrete timestep, they remain easy to compute as dynamical systems.

Results and conclusion

The authors describe a set of experiments where changes in concentrations of certain proteins involved in the reactions, in addition to external stimuli, could affect the onset of apoptosis. The CA simulated the complex reaction pathways that could determine the fate of the cell. It was found that a delicate equilibrium existed between several proteins which could be perturbed by external factors which in turn determined whether apoptosis took place. Readers are directed to Siehs *et al.* (2002) for more information on the results obtained from these experiments.

In summary, these experiments confirmed what was known experimentally and replicated expected results for different sets of stimuli and protein concentrations. Again, this work could be used to simulate the process of apoptosis under a number of different, artificial conditions, with a small computational requirement. The authors set up the registers and steps in such a way that this approach could be used to model any number of molecular reactions and therefore could be used to simulate a large number of intracellular processes.

Conclusions

The above work showed the simulations of systems that are possible with CA. The main aim of this research was to investigate the behaviour of molecules in highly complex environments where there might be many hundreds or thousands of molecules interacting at once. It is in this application area where CA can excel and is mainly due to their parallel nature, in that all the parameters are updated in one discrete timestep for every element of the grid. This not only allows the processes to be observed at specified time intervals, but also provides the opportunity to simulate systems on parallel hardware and thereby increase performance in comparison to similar sequential techniques.

10.4 Background

Cellular automata were conceived in the late 1940s, making them one of the oldest techniques in this book. They were introduced by John von

Neumann on the suggestion of Stan Ulam to provide a more realistic model for complex systems. In fact von Neumann, in addition to being a physicist and mathematician, was actually more interested in the reductionist biological applications seen in this book. Since their inception, CA have been used in many of the 'hard science' fields such as physics and fluid dynamics, as well as fascinating mathematicians. So while they maintain a pedigree of being highly intertwined with biology from the very beginning, they have perhaps not been used as much as would have been expected in the recent explosion in bioinformatics applications.

10.5 Summary of chapter

1 Cellular automata consist of a grid of cells which can adopt a number of states.

2 Cells change states by virtue of a set of state transition rules which are applied in discrete time.

3 Cellular automata can be thought of as stylized universes, repeatedly applying the laws of the universe to the elements within it.

4 The behaviour of a CA is deterministic, but the outcome of applying a set of rules to an initial random starting point can be difficult to predict.

5 Applications in bioinformatics are relatively few and tend to be restricted to the simulation of phenomena rather than the optimization of systems in biology. Nevertheless they have found a number of applications in bioinformatics.

10.6 References and further reading

Holland, J.H. (1998) *Emergence: From Chaos to Order.* Oxford University Press, Oxford, UK.

Keedwell, E.C. and Khu, S.T. (2005) A novel cellular-automaton inspired approach to optimal water distribution network design *ASCE Journal of Computing in Civil Engineering*, in press.

Kier, L.B., Cheng, C.K., Testa, B. *et al.* (1996) A cellular automata model of enzyme kinetics. *Journal of Molecular Graphics*, **14**, 227–231.

Siehs, C., Oberbauer, R., Mayer, G. *et al.* (2002) Discrete simulation of homo- and heterodimerization in the apoptosis affector phase. *Bioinformatics*, **18**, 67–76.

Toffoli, T. and Margolus, N. (1987) *Cellular Automata Machines: A New Environment for Modelling*, MIT Press, Cambridge, Massachussetts.

Wolfram, S. (1984) Cellular automata as models of complexity. *Nature*, **311** (4), 419–424.

11
Hybrid Methods

11.1 Method

The intelligent methods shown throughout this book have demonstrated that they can each individually be used to find interesting solutions to bioinformatics problems. However, occasionally one technique will not be sufficient to solve a problem, often due to the nature of the problem or because no one algorithm fits the problem requirements. In this instance two or more machine learning techniques can be combined together to create hybrids which can make use of the attributes of each algorithm in such a way that they are more successful at solving the problem. These hybrid algorithms are often experimental in nature because they are created to solve a specific need in the field of biology. This also means that they are often created for a specific purpose, and this approach differs from the more generic methods in this book as hybrids tend to be highly tuned to the problem they were designed to solve and means that they can often outperform the single algorithms from which they are derived. Hybrid algorithms are known under a variety of names: *memetic algorithms*, for instance, relate to evolutionary-based hybrid algorithms in combination with local search techniques such as hill-climbing.

There are no hard and fast rules dictating which algorithms can be combined to give a hybrid, but as will be seen later, evolutionary methods are often favoured because they can be hybridized in a number of ways.

1 The mutation or crossover operations can be implemented differently with other algorithms. For instance the mutation operator can be replaced with a local search algorithm.

Intelligent Bioinformatics   Edward Keedwell and Ajit Narayanan
© 2005 John Wiley & Sons, Ltd

2   The objective function can be used to compute the result of other algorithms. For instance, the GA can create a structure which is then used to set the parameters for a neural network, from which the fitness is returned.

3   The genetic search can be interleaved with other algorithms. For instance, the GA can be run for a number of generations and then stopped to allow a local search to take place. These solutions can then be used by the GA in the subsequent optimization.

These three methods are good examples of how hybrids are constructed where evolutionary methods are concerned. It should be noted that they differ in interaction in that the first method above can be thought of as tightly coupled: both algorithms' execution is intertwined. The second method is less tightly coupled: only the objective function links the two. Nevertheless, the secondary algorithm is called for every solution evaluation. The final method is loosely coupled, since the algorithms do not have any direct interaction with each other; rather, they are executed in relative isolation. Evolutionary hybrids can make use of a variety of schemes for hybridization and this explains their popularity in this domain. These examples give an idea of the hybrids that can be created between different algorithms and approaches, and essentially there is no limit to the types and methods of creating a combination of two or more artificial intelligence algorithms.

The next few sections describe hybrid approaches and the problems they are designed to solve. This is in contrast to the other technique chapters in this book which maintain a distinction between technique and application and is necessary because hybrids and the problems they solve are often closely linked.

11.2 Neural-genetic algorithm for analysing gene expression data

The problems of gene expression analysis have been described in some detail previously in this book, so a short explanation will suffice here. Currently there are two types of microarray experimentation that are attracting interest in the literature: temporal analysis involves exploring the interactions of genes over time, and classification analysis attempts to discover those genes or groups of genes that are associated with a class value. The two analyses are driven by the goals of the experiment and the type of microarray experiments that have been performed by the biologist. This, in turn, dictates the type and scale of microarray data which is available for bioinformaticians to use.

Temporal analysis

Temporal analysis consists of a number of microarray samples over time, normally taken from a single organism exposed to a variety of conditions to assess the genetic response to those conditions. The task in such experiments is to determine the interactions between genes or clusters of genes over time. It is widely acknowledged that a large portion of genetic activity is self-regulated, in that the proteins created by the expression of certain genes themselves cause other genes to be expressed in this cell. The goal of the analysis is to determine these complex regulatory connections from small-scale and large-scale expression data.

Classification analysis

The classification analysis consists of a number of microarray samples taken from a number of individual organisms (often patients diagnosed with a disease). Each of the samples has a class associated with it which is independently assigned. The majority of classification studies are performed on human subjects in an attempt to discover the genetic differences between, say, patients with cancer and those without. Classifications can either be determined by a medical diagnosis, or in cases where the diagnosis is very difficult, the pathology of the disease. There are some difficulties with this approach, namely, that the classification by humans in some cases is not guaranteed to be correct, and also that significant genetic patterns are not guaranteed to cause the cancer – they could be symptoms. Despite this, analysis of classificatory microarray data is one of the most popular activities in bioinformatics as the number of gene expression databases, taken from microarray experiments, which are available on the web increases.[1]

Neural-genetic approach

Chapter 8 describes a standard GA approach to the problem of extracting regulatory networks from microarray data, but there are some difficulties

[1] See http://www.broad.mit.edu/cancer/ for some example data-sets.

with the approach. Experiments conducted in Keedwell (2003) showed that the approach of generating an entire regulatory network by GA was not feasible for the size of real-world networks. This was because in a matrix representation any gene could potentially regulate any other and so the size of the network was the square of the number of genes. For a network matrix of even 1000 genes, this led to a chromosome size of 1 000 000 integers, which was too large for most GA software, and would require excessive computation to evaluate. Although the premise that any gene can affect any other in the network must be maintained, biology and complexity analysis tell us that the actual number of genes which can regulate another is likely to be smaller than six (details can be seen in Keedwell, 2003). Therefore this restriction can reduce the complexity of the genetic approach by maintaining a distinction between the regulating and regulated genes in the data-set. Each regulated gene value at time $t = 1$ must be considered as some combination of, at most, six regulating genes at time $t = 0$. By using the GA to evaluate each regulated gene in turn rather than the entire set, the chromosome size is reduced to a maximum of six integers for each regulated gene. The optimization for a regulated gene takes place until such time as a satisfactorily low error is achieved or a limit on the number of iterations is reached. The algorithm then moves to the next regulated gene in the network, and the process is repeated. This occurs, in turn for all genes in the network, which therefore allows running times to increase linearly with respect to the number of genes considered.

So far, the approach uses only the GA, but there is a difficulty with using solely GAs in this approach. Experiments were conducted on the rat spinal cord dataset (Spellman *et al.*, 1998) where the output of the generated network was compared with the actual gene expression data. It was shown that, while the GA performed well initially with a good decrease in error, as the optimization progressed and the genetic algorithm began to converge, the error would stop at levels as high as 16 per cent. It was considered at this point that the combination and generation of new weights in the network was the problem. The GA was quickly finding a set of genes, but the floating point weights that were generated were being optimized very slowly. Therefore another method was considered to generate the weights for the network, namely, the gradient descent method employed in neural networks. The gradient descent algorithm was well-suited to minimizing the difference between two sets of floating-point variables, and the weights could be added to the network structure. This 'neural-genetic' approach made use of the attributes of both algorithms. The GA was used to discover those genes that were important in the

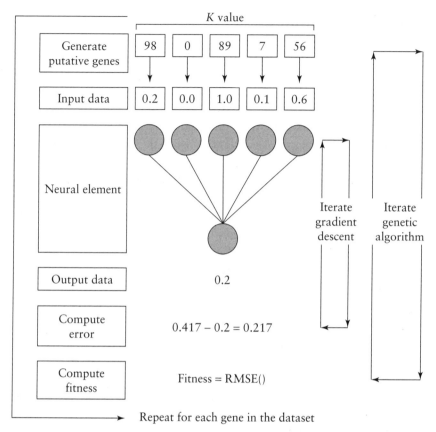

Figure 11.1 The execution of the neural-genetic approach (RMSE = root mean squared error)

regulation of the gene in question in an efficient manner, whereas the neural network was used to minimize the difference between the input of the genes selected and the expression levels of the regulated gene quickly. Figure 11.1 shows the architecture of the hybrid neural-genetic approach. The GA chromosome finds a set of candidate genes for regulation of the current regulated gene. This data is then selected from the data base and the neural network is used to minimize the difference between the regulating genes and the regulated gene output. The error from the neural network is then returned to the GA as the fitness of the chromosome. The GA can then use the genetic operators to discover more optimal sets of genes. In this way, both those important genes and the weights for those genes for entry into the regulatory network can be determined.

The technique used the sigmoid function backpropagation equations as described in Chapter 7 and was trained on the rat spinal cord dataset which consists of 112 genes over eight timesteps taken from the spinal cord during the development of the rat. Using a k-value of four (restricting the genetic algorithm to a maximum of four genes to regulate any other gene), the resulting network was able to reproduce the training data to some 97.6 per cent accuracy. This experiment suggested that the neural-genetic approach was capable of extracting regulatory interactions from microarray time series data with efficiency and that it could discover networks from gene expression data consisting of thousands of genes within a few hours. Additional experiments on artificial time series data showed that it could discover gene interactions that were embedded in Boolean data.

The approach can also be used for classification analysis with only some minor modifications. In some ways, a classification problem can be seen as a similar problem to that of regulation in that a set of genes must be discovered which account for the variation in classification, much the same way as they must be discovered to determine the variation in a gene value. Therefore a 'network' can be created which links a set of genes with the classification (i.e. 'diseased' or 'not diseased'). However, the classification normally consists of a small set of possible values, and these can be decomposed into a set of binary attributes.

Table 11.1 shows the conversion process from three discrete classes to the field representation. Each potential class has a space in the field which takes the value 1 if the class is selected and 0 otherwise. When combined with the absence–presence model given as an option in most gene expression datasets, the algorithm can be used to find those genes which are 'regulating' the classification shown in the training data. In addition to this, some minor changes are required to the backpropagation component to reduce the granularity of the weights that are discovered in comparison with the approach used for regulatory networks. This is due to the fact that floating-point weightings for attributes do not make sense for classification in the same way as they do for regulatory

Table 11.1 Conversion of classes into enumerations and then a field representation

Classification	Enumeration	Conversio
Acute lymphoblastic leukaemia	1	1,0,0
Acute myeloid leukaemia	2	0,1,0
Unknown	3	0,0,1

networks. To achieve this increased granularity, the neural network uses the step function rather than the sigmoid function used in the regulatory networks. The result is a rule which classifies a single class by naming a number of attributes and associated weights for each attribute. This allows a number of attributes (genes) to be involved in the classification, but weighted according to their influence. A large number of candidate rules are generated during the optimization process, so the final rule is selected firstly according to accuracy, then by parsimony and finally by test accuracy.

An example of the rules generated by this approach on the multiple myeloma dataset can be seen here.

```
Rule: 537
L18972_at_AC = P -2
X16416_at_AC = P -3
X16832_at_AC = P 2
X57129_at_AC = A 3
L36033_at_AC = A -3
      -> normal
0/22
TestError: 1:9

Rule: 2796
M63928_at_AC = P -2
X16416_at_AC = P 3
U40490_at_AC = A 1
M33195_at_AC = P -1
L36033_at_AC = A 2
      -> myeloma
0/42
TestError: 1:31
```

where A = absent and P = present. Therefore a positive weight indicates that this attribute in its indicated state (present or absent) is required to classify the data. Larger weights indicate more influence on the classification of the dataset. The figures after each rule indicate that they classify the training data with no misclassifications, but that one case in each of the test sets is misclassified. This result was considerably better than that discovered by See5 on the same dataset, although only the standard options were used. More results on a variety of datasets can be found in Keedwell (2003), including an investigation into the biological plausibility of a variety of the discovered genes.

Conclusions

The advantages of combining the GA and the neural network in this manner are the speed of execution and the flexibility of the final solutions generated by the algorithm. By generating a segment of the regulatory network for each regulated gene in turn, the GA can concentrate on discovering the correct combination of genes and the neural element effectively minimizes the difference between the expression values of each of the genes. An additional feature of this approach is that the regulation of single genes can be determined in isolation, if required, yielding the possibility of just-in-time regulation discovery. A biologist may be interested in the regulatory interactions of a handful of genes, and this technique would allow the biologist to select those genes of interest as well as execute the algorithm on just those of concern. The approach uses the current biological constraints, namely, the necessary sparsity of gene regulator networks, to its advantage. Both elements of the technique are limited: the GA by the k-value and the neural network by a maximum weight value. This goes some way towards ensuring that a sub-optimal selection of genes cannot be compensated for by the selection of weights. The flexibility of this approach is shown in that, by making these small adjustments, the neural-genetic model can be converted to operate either on temporal or classificatory data. The resulting weighted classification models are unusual in their make-up but provide the biologist with some notion of the importance of each of the genes in classification. This is not normally the case with decision tree or other classification algorithms. The neural-genetic approach shows the advantage of combining two algorithms that have contrasting properties for the study of microarray data.

11.3 Genetic algorithm and *k* nearest neighbour hybrid for biochemistry solvation

A further GA-based technique, the work of Peterson, Doom and Raymer (2004), considered the use of a hybrid of a standard GA (discussed in Chapter 8 of this book) and a k nearest neighbour technique (discussed in Chapter 5). This approach was applied to the problem of classifying water molecules according to whether they were displaced when a ligand (such as a drug or other molecule) attached itself to the surface of the protein. Therefore extracting meaningful, accurate knowledge about this problem could provide an insight into the behaviour of drugs when binding to the protein surface that could assist drug designers.

GA-Knn method

The genetic algorithm k nearest neighbour (GA-Knn) method makes use of a cosine-based Knn classification. This is slightly different from normal Knn classification in that each of the features in the data-set is weighted and the final classification predicted by the system for a new example is the sum of those weights. In this two-class example, a positive sum indicates one class and a negative sum, another. These weights are optimized by the GA by using the first N (where N is the number of features) elements of the chromosome to evolve the weights for classification. This constitutes the first section of optimization for the technique. The second N points of the chromosome are involved with changing the point of origin for the Knn classifier. When predicting the class of a new solution, the Knn classifier compute the 'nearest neighbour' based on the angle created when plotting a solution in two feature dimensions, between the origin and the test point. The similarity between the angle of the test point and points in the training set determines the nearest neighbour classification. However, if the origin is changed in one or both axes, a more optimal set of neighbours could be found. This constitutes the second part of the chromosome, where N points determine the offset of the origin for each feature. Finally, the k value for the Knn classifier is determined as a single integer at the end of the chromosome. Therefore the GA is involved with optimizing the weight, offset and k values for the cosine-based Knn classifier.

Classification results

The authors compared their technique against a suite of other techniques known as WEKA (including decision tree, neural network and rule induction algorithms) on the problem of ligand-binding water conservation. The GA-Knn hybrid method was compared with the WEKA methods by determining the accuracy of the top three runs of the method in comparison with the top three techniques taken from the WEKA suite on the water conservation dataset. The dataset itself contained 5542 water molecules of which 3405 were conserved when the ligand docked and 2137 were displaced, taken from measurements of 30 separate proteins. Each water molecule was represented by eight measured features:

1 the number of protein atoms which surrounded the water molecule,

2 the frequency with which the atoms surrounding the water molecule were found to bind to water molecules in another database of proteins,

3 thermal mobility,

4 the number of hydrogen bonds between the water molecule and the protein,

5 the number of hydrogen bonds to other water molecules, and

6,7 and 8 three additional temperature factors of either the molecule itself or the neighbouring atoms.

The task for the algorithm was to distinguish between those molecules that would be displaced or conserved when a ligand binds, based on these eight measurements of the water molecule itself.

In addition to the accuracy percentage from the experiment, the authors also recorded the balance of the classification. Many techniques classify one class with greater accuracy than the others by concentrating on the most frequent class. This approach often yields information of limited use, since the more frequent class was also often the least interesting. (This had been noted especially in areas such as credit-risk analysis where the vast majority of credit card holders were trustworthy and constituted the larger class, whereas the company wished to identify the credit-risks.) The balance measure was designed to rate the classification according to how well balanced the classification was over all the classes. The top three GA-Knn runs achieved accuracy similar to those from the WEKA model (between 64 and 66 per cent), but with much better balance, indicating that the interactions discovered by GA-Knn were more interesting. These results showed that the important features that were weighted most strongly by the GA-Knn classifier were those which related to the thermal mobility of the molecules.

Conclusion

This study provided a good example of how GAs could be combined with another technique to produce good classification results both in the accuracy and transparency of the obtained results. This application differed from the neural-genetic approach described above in that the GA was used to modify the parameters of a standard classification technique. The hybridization of the two algorithms aims for the GA to pick good weight and offset sets for the Knn to use and classify the examples. The GA could be viewed as 'tuning' the parameters of the classifier whereas in the neural-genetic approach it was directly involved in the knowledge discovery process. The results shown by Peterson, Doom and Raymer (2004) were encouraging, especially in that the classification was well balanced. The balance of the final classification was all-important in datasets where the two classes were not equally represented – quite often the case in real-world problems including those in bioinformatics. Finally, while the accuracy was similar between this and the established techniques, the WEKA system used a cross-validation technique (see Chapter 5 for more on this), whereas the GA-Knn approach was evaluated using bootstrapped data. The accuracy of bootstrapped data can be different from that where a test-set is used (either in cross-validation or standard testing), as the same example can appear numerous times in each dataset. Still, this example neatly showed the advantages of using a hybrid system for a specific and pressing problem in bioinformatics.

11.4 Genetic programming neural networks for determining gene – gene interactions in epidemiology

This approach by Ritchie *et al.* (2003, 2004) combines two techniques seen separately in other chapters of this book. Genetic programming (described in Chapter 9) is combined with neural network theory (Chapter 7) to predict the probability of disease based on the observed genetics of individuals with and without the disease. This study is different from those described above in that the data is entirely artificial. No real biological data is used to validate the model, but the principles used in generating the data do have biological plausible roots. The approach highlights yet another useful combination of techniques.

Genetic programming neural networks (GPNN)

Originally suggested by Koza and Rice (1991), GP neural networks combine the functional optimization methodology of GP but within stricter bounds than normal. Standard GP, without restriction, can evolve any set of operators and terminals that satisfy the problem, although often restrictions are placed on the total size of the tree that can be created (to restrict *bloat*). However, GPNN restricts the type of structure which can be evolved, rather than the size, so that the final tree resembles a standard neural network. The operators are determined as a weighting function and an activation function. In addition to this, the terminal set is defined as a set of floating-point values (for use in the operator functions) and the input variables gained from the database. The restrictions placed on the GP ensure that the root node always represents the output of the neural network, and that an activation function and weighting functions must directly descend from the root node. Beyond this, however, the algorithm is free to select from the operator and terminal set. This allows the GP element to optimize a neural network structure that minimizes the difference between output and desired response. There is no requirement for the network to use backpropagation or any other gradient descent learning method to determine the weights in the network, as these are determined during the optimization process.

Discovering gene-gene interactions in simulated data

The authors used their approach to determine, from a set of single-nucleotide-polymorphisms (SNPs), those functional polymorphisms which are implicated in a particular disease. The data is simulated so that each of the 400 data records (constituting 200 cases of the 'disease' and 200 controls) contains two or three functional polymorphisms and a further eight or nine polymorphisms to make 10 for each record. The probability of developing the disease is reflected by using a table of penetrance function values. All of the data in the experiment requires that at least two of the polymorphisms interacted with each other to create increased susceptibility to disease. None of the effects seen in the data could be determined solely by a main effect of one of the genes. The authors state that this was particularly important for epistasis studies where genes had little or no effect by themselves, but individuals who possessed a certain pairing, or combination, of genes drastically increased their chance of developing the disease.

A 10-fold cross-validation approach was used to determine the performance of GPNN on the data. This involved generating 10 datasets, training the approach on nine of them and then testing on the remaining one. This was repeated for the 10 possible combinations of training and test sets. The task for the GPNN model is to determine the interaction of the genes that have a combined effect and yield a diseased or non-diseased individual to a greater or lesser degree depending on the heritability of the genes. The authors computed 'power' to be the number of times the correct SNPs were discovered with greater cross-validation consistency than the other SNPs in the dataset. The GPNN approach was applied to a number of datasets, with a varying number of genes, allele frequencies and heritability scores. These 20 datasets give a good cross section of the possible datasets as each of the significant parameters is modified systematically. As would be expected, the performance of the GPNN is dependent on the type of model used to generate the data. The GPNN solutions varied from 100 per cent to 1 per cent over 20 datasets, whereas the performance for the comparison technique, stepwise logistic regression was 0 per cent in all cases. The GPNN approach appears to be significantly more capable in determining which SNPs were responsible for the disease under a number of conditions.

The GPNN approach was able to extract the functional polymorphisms from the data, dependent on the level of effect seen in the phenotype (this was denoted as heritability). The comparison technique, stepwise linear regression, was unable to determine any of the functional groups over the dataset.

Conclusions

The GPNN technique had been shown to accurately extract, for a certain dataset, the functionally active SNPs from artificial data which had been created to closely resemble biological data. The approach made use of the ability of GP to discover good near-optimal solutions for this problem. However, the reasons behind the use of GP *neural networks* is never described beyond the fact that other researchers had used neural networks for this task. There appeared to be no problem-specific reason for the GP method to be restricted to a neural network style representation, as the neural network approach could prove to be more restrictive than simply using genetic programming. Also, the choice of comparison technique, in stepwise logistic regression (which failed to determine any of the functional polymorphisms) did not appear to validate the GPNN approach greatly, although the authors stated that it was frequently applied in the field of human genetics. A favourable comparison of the hybrid technique with either of the established single techniques could perhaps enhance this application and the idea of GPNN. However, this application did show a further successful hybrid technique which delivered improved results over the currently used method.

11.5 Application guidelines

Hybrid techniques are not necessary, or even desirable, for all bioinformatics applications. As described previously, the loss of generality when considering a hybrid means that any advances gained in the application may not be applicable to other problem domains. Typically, hybrids are constructed where one algorithm is lacking in some respect and another can be used to compensate for this shortfall. For instance, the computational requirement for genetic algorithms to find an optimal set of floating-point values is often far greater than that required by a neural network so a hybrid may be beneficial. Similarly, a neural network structure is difficult to interpret whereas a GA chromosome, generally speaking, is not and therefore this property may be an advantage. In general then, the application itself must drive the use of a hybrid algorithm, in that the computational capability or need for transparency of the problem exerts demands that one single algorithm cannot meet.

11.6 Conclusions

The hybrids shown in this chapter all include some element of evolutionary computation and this is because they naturally lend themselves to being part of a hybrid. As described earlier, the flexibility of evolutionary computing makes these algorithms favourable to hybridization. In addition to this, they make use of a symbolic representation, and efficiently utilize the computing resources available.

The above approaches have shown that there are a practically limitless number of ways in which the intelligent approaches described in this book can be combined. The hybrids shown here often outperform their single-algorithm counterparts, or are more applicable to the bioinformatics problem being solved. This increase in performance though is often tempered by the fact that the nature of hybrid algorithms, and particularly their high degree of specialization, mean that the problem-independence which the single techniques possess does not transfer to the hybrid technology. Nevertheless, hybrid approaches are becoming more and more popular as the number of researchers using the standard techniques increases.

11.7 Summary of chapter

1 Hybrid algorithms can be used to solve a variety of problems in bioinformatics.

2 The hybrid algorithm often improves on either a single algorithm, in terms of performance, or in the transparency of its results.

3 There are numerous ways in which algorithms can be combined, but the method selected is often determined by the problem formulation.

4 Evolutionary algorithms are popular for constructing hybrid models due to the ease with which they can be combined with other methods.

11.8 References and further reading

Keedwell, E. (2003) *Knowledge Discovery from Gene Expression Data Using Neural-Genetic Models*, PhD Thesis, University of Exeter, Exeter, UK. Available from http://www.ex.ac.uk/~eckeedwe.

Keedwell, E. and Narayanan, A. (2003) Genetic algorithms for gene expression analysis, in *Applications of Evolutionary Computing LNCS 2611* (eds G. Raidl *et al.*). Proceedings of EvoBIO2003 1st European Workshop on Evolutionary Bioinformatics, pp. 76–86.

Koza, J.R. and Rice, J.P. (1991) *Genetic Generation of Both the Weights and Architecture for a Neural Network*. IEEE International Joint Conference on Neural Networks, 1991, Vol II, pp. 397–404.

Peterson, M., Doom, T. and Raymer, M. (2004) "GA-facilitated knowledge discovery and pattern recognition optimization applied to the biochemistry of protein solvation" *Proceedings of ACM Genetic and Evolutionary Computation Conference* (GECCO) 2004, Seattle WA, pp. 426–437, June 2004.

Ritchie, M.D., White, W.C, Parker, J.S. *et al.* (2003) Optimization of neural network architecture using genetic programming improves detection and modeling of gene–gene interactions in studies of human diseases. *BMC Bioinformatics 2003*, Vol. 4. Available from http://www.biomedcentral.com/1471-2105/4/28.

Ritchie, M.D., Coffey, C.S. and Moore, J.H. (2004) *Genetic Programming Neural Networks as a Bioinformatics Tool for Human Genetics.* Proceedings of the Genetic and Evolutionary Computation Conference (GECCO 04), in *Lecture Notes in Computer Science 3012 (LNCS 3012)* (eds Deb *et al.*) Vol 2, pp. 438–448, Springer.

Spellman, P., Sherlock, G., Zhang, M. *et al.* (1998) Comprehensive identification of cell cycle-regulated genes of the yeast Saccharomyces cerevisial by microarray hybridization. *Mol. Biol. Cell,* **9,** 3273–3297.

Index

Note: Figures and Tables are indicated by *italic page numbers*, footnotes by suffix 'n'

"...Having the whole of functional genomics/proteomics in one place will be very attractive..."

Ian Dunham, Wellcome Trust Sanger Institute, UK

Encyclopedia of

Genetics, Genomics, Proteomics and Bioinformatics

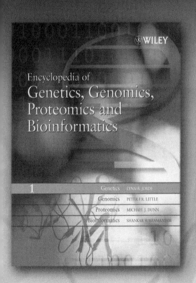

Edited by

LYNN B. JORDE,

PETER F. R. LITTLE,

MICHAEL J. DUNN

and

SHANKAR SUBRAMANIAM

The *Encyclopedia of Genetics, Genomics, Proteomics and Bioinformatics* brings together the latest advances in these dynamic and rapidly growing fields and ensures a truly multidisciplinary approach. The focus is on human and mouse genomes, but other important model eukaryotes, and pathogenic bacteria, are given in-depth coverage.

Available in full colour print and online
via Wiley InterScience®

0-470-84974-6   October 2005   8 Volume Set

Visit www.wiley.com for details

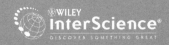